CANCER CARE STANDARDS

CANCER CARE STANDARDS

Putting the Puzzle Pieces Together
to Personalize Medicine

COLLEEN O. LEE
www.lee-medical.com

ISBN-13: 9781482518207
ISBN-10: 1482518201
Library of Congress Control Number: 2015902573
CreateSpace Independent Publishing Platform
North Charleston, South Carolina

DEDICATION

To my family who has witnessed and endured many lives
affected by cancer and emerged more appreciative of
health and in vibrant pursuit in enjoying life to its fullest.

DISCLAIMER

This book is intended to serve solely as a resource guide for health professionals, patients and caregivers, and cancer care advocates. It is not intended to replace the care of a health care provider, genetic counselor, or oncologist.

CONTENTS

TABLES

ACKNOWLEDGMENTS

I would like to acknowledge my family and friends for their continued, meaningful encouragement in the writing of this book and in support of my many eclectic professional adventures.

"This is a time of extraordinary change and opportunity in cancer care."

American Society for Clinical Oncology
The State of Cancer Care in America: 2014™
Executive Summary

§

The number of older adults in the US will double between 2010 and 2030. This doubling will lead to a 30% increase in the number of cancer survivors and a 45% increase in the incidence of cancer.

Institute of Medicine of the National Academies
Delivering High-Quality Cancer Care: Charting a New Course for a System in Crisis, 2013, p. 2

§

"Thanks to research, Americans today are more likely to survive a cancer diagnosis and enjoy a higher quality of life than at any other time in history."

American Association for Cancer Research
2014 Cancer Progress Report: Research is Transforming Lives

1

CANCER FUNDAMENTALS:
IT ALL STARTS WITH THE CELL

WHAT IS CANCER AND HOW
DOES IT DEVELOP?

Cancer is a term for diseases in which abnormal cells divide without control and may occupy nearby tissues in the body (National Cancer Institute (NCI, 2014). Cancer is simply not one disease but many diseases. There are more than 100 different kinds of cancer.

All cancers begin in the body's basic unit of life – the cell. The human body is composed of many types of cells. These cells grow and divide in a well-ordered fashion to produce more cells as needed to keep the body functioning in a healthy manner. As a cell becomes old or damaged, it dies and is replaced with a new cell.

Sometimes this orderly process does not occur as planned. The genetic material of a cell, known as DNA (deoxyribonucleic acid), may turn out to be changed or damaged, creating changes or mutations that affect normal cell growth, development, and division. When this occurs, cells do not die when they should and new cells develop when the body does not need them. The extra new cells may form a group or mass of tissue called a tumor.

A tumor may be one of two types: benign (noncancerous) or malignant (cancerous). Benign tumors, when removed, often do not recur nor do they spread to other parts of the body. On the other hand, malignant (cancerous) tumors may spread to nearby tissues and organs as well as other parts of the body. Metastasis is the term used to describe when cancer cells spread from one part of the body to another. When the cells from the primary cancer are found in another part of the body, it is called metastatic cancer by the primary site's location. For example, if a skin cancer like melanoma spread to a distant organ such as the liver, it would be called metastatic melanoma versus liver cancer. Not all cancers form tumors. Examples are leukemia, lymphoma, and multiple myeloma. Leukemia is a cancer of the bone marrow and blood. Lymphoma is a cancer of lymphocytes (a type of white blood cell). Multiple myeloma is a cancer of the plasma cells (also a type of white blood cell). Some refer to these types of cancer as "liquid" tumors.

WHAT ARE CANCER SUBTYPES?

Most cancers are named for the type of cell or bodily organ from which they originate and develop. Cancer subtypes are the smaller groups that a type of cancer can be divided into, based on certain features of the cells. These features include how the cancer cells appear under a microscope and whether there are certain substances in or on the cells or certain changes to the DNA in the cell. Knowing the subtype of a cancer is essential in planning the course of treatment and developing a prognosis or clinical outcome (NCI, 2014).

WHAT CAUSES CANCER?

The causes of cancer are numerous with some causes being unavoidable and others being avoidable. Some causes of certain cancers are known and other causes remain unknown at the present. Several unavoidable causes or risk factors for the development of some types of cancer are increasing age and family history of cancer. Several avoidable causes or risk factors for the development of some types of cancer are tobacco products, sunlight (ultraviolet light), ionizing radiation, poor diet, alcohol, lack of exercise, increased body weight, certain chemicals, viruses, bacteria, and hormones (NCI, 2014). While there are known and unknown risk factors, a key principle is that having one or more risk factors *doesn't mean* that one will develop cancer. Most people with one or more risk factors for cancer *do not ever* develop cancer.

What is a 'lifetime risk' or 'relative risk'?

The term 'risk' refers to, most often, a lifetime risk or relative risk. 'Lifetime risk' is the probability that an individual will develop or die from cancer over his or her lifetime. Estimates of risk are based on the 'average' experience of the general population and may not be directly related to the risk of an individual (because of differences in exposure or family history, for example).

'Relative risk' measures the strength of the relationship between a single risk factor and the developing of a certain type of cancer. The basis of the comparison is between those who have a risk factor compared to those who do not have this risk factor.

Common cancer risk factors and reasons for these risk factors are listed in **Table 1 (NCI, 2014)**.

Table 1. Cancer Risk Factors and Reasons for Risk	
Risk Factor	*Reason for Risk*
Increasing age	Most cancers occur in people over the age of 65 years.
Family History of Cancer	A few genetic mutations are passed down through families.
Tobacco	Tobacco products contain some chemicals that are known causes of cancer. Exposure may be self-exposure (firsthand), secondhand smoke, and smokeless tobacco.

Sunlight [Ultraviolet (UV)]	UV radiation from the sun, sunlamps, and tanning booths causes early aging and skin damage that can lead to skin cancers.
Ionizing radiation	Radioactive gases like radon, radioactive fallout from a nuclear event, radiation emitted via x-rays and radiation therapy to treat cancer can cause cell damage that leads to cancer.
Poor diet, Lack of exercise, Increased body weight	Diets high in fat intake, inactivity, and increased in body weight due to poor diet and lack of activity may impact the body's ability to fight some diseases including cancer.
Alcohol	For women who have more than 1-2 drinks per day and for men who have more than 2-4 drinks per day have increased risks of cancer due to changes in cells making up mucous membranes.
Chemicals	Exposure to chemicals such as asbestos, benzene, benzidine, cadmium, nickel, or vinyl chloride in the workplace can cause cancer.
Viruses	Infection with certain viruses may increase the risk for developing cancer. Examples include: human papillomavirus (HPV), human immunodeficiency virus (HIV), hepatitis B virus and hepatitis C virus.
Bacteria	Infection with certain bacteria may increase the risk for developing cancer. An example is helicobacter pylori (H. pylori)
Hormones	Exposure to some forms of estrogen such as DES (diethylstilbestrol) may lead to the development of cancer. Estrogen- products (alone or in combination) for the treatment of menopausal symptoms may increase the risk for health conditions including cancer.

CANCER TYPES

WHAT ARE THE MOST COMMON CANCER TYPES?

Cancer types that are referred to as 'common' are those identified with the greatest frequency in the United States (US). The incidence rate to meet the requirements as a 'common' cancer is greater than 40,000 new cases. Currently, the most common cancers in alphabetical order are listed in **Table 2** (American Cancer Society (ACS, 2014).

Table 2. Common Cancer Types
Bladder
Breast
Colon & Rectal
Endometrial
Kidney
Leukemia
Lung
Melanoma
Non-Hodgkin Lymphoma
Pancreatic
Thyroid

ARE THERE DIFFERENCES IN CANCER OCCURRENCE BY GENDER?

In the US, there are gender differences related to the occurrence of cancer. For example, the lifetime risk of a male developing cancer is a little less than a 1 in 2 risk. In women, the risk of developing cancer is slightly more than in 1 in 3. A comparison of leading cancer types by gender are listed in **Table 3** (ACS, 2014).

Table 3. Leading Cancer Types by Gender	
Male	*Female*
Prostate	Breast
Lung & bronchus	Lung & bronchus
Colon & rectum	Colon & rectum
Urinary Bladder	Uterine corpus
Melanoma of the skin	Thyroid
Kidney & renal pelvis	Non-Hodgkin lymphoma
Non-Hodgkin lymphoma	Melanoma of the skin
Oral cavity & pharynx	Kidney & renal pelvis
Leukemia	Pancreas
Pancreas	Ovary

WHAT ARE THE TISSUE TYPES FROM WHICH CANCER CAN DEVELOP?

- Carcinomas are the most common types of cancer and arise from cells that cover the internal and external and body surfaces. Examples of carcinomas are lung, breast, and colon cancer.
- Sarcomas are cancers that arise from cells found in the supporting tissues of the body such as bone, cartilage, fat, connective tissue, and muscle.
- Lymphomas are cancers that arise in the tissue and lymph nodes of the immune system in the body.
- Leukemias are cancers of the blood cells that grow in the bone marrow and spread to the bloodstream.

HOW ARE CANCERS NAMED?

Cancers are named from the type of tissue from which they arise using common prefixes. Examples are listed in **Table 4**.

Table 4. Naming of Cancers by Tissue Type	
Common Prefix	*Cell/Tissue/Organ*
Adeno-	Gland
Hepato-	Liver
Lympho-	Lymphocyte
Melano-	Pigmented cell (skin)
Osteo-	Bone

WHICH CANCERS ARE CONSIDERED TO BE THE MOST RARE?

Rare cancers (also known as cancers of rare sites) are those which occur in 2000 or less cases per year in the US. It is not clear as to why there are certain body sites in which rare cancers arise. Examples are listed in **Table 5.**

Table 5. Rare Cancers in the US	
Cases Per Year	*Primary Site*
1000-2000	Nasal Cavity Merkel Cell Invasive Male Breast Cancer
500-1000	Trachea, Mediastinum Papillary Serous Cystadenocarcinoma (of the peritoneum) Squamous Cell Carcinoma of the Penis
250-500	Trachea Germ Cell of the Mediastinum Sweat Gland Adenocarcinoma Sebaceous Adenocarcinoma
<250	Squamous Cell Carcinoma of the Trachea Cancer of the Middle Ear Female Ligaments and Adnexa Squamous Cell Carcinoma of the Scrotum Paget Disease of the Scrotum

Adapted from NCI, SEER Survival Monograph Table 30.1 Cancers of rate sites: Number and Distribution of Cases by Primary Site, Sex, Race, and SEER Summary

§

References

American Cancer Society, *Cancer Facts & Figures 2014* http://www.cancer.org/acs/groups/content/@research/ documents/webcontent/acspc-042151.pdf
National Cancer Institute
    What is Cancer? http://www.cancer.gov/ cancertopics/cancerlibrary/what-is-cancer
    Cancer Causes and Risk Factors http://www.cancer. gov/cancertopics/causes
    Surveillance, Epidemiology, and End Results Program http://seer.cancer.gov/statistics/summaries. html

2

Cancer Continuum: Screening

What is the cancer continuum?

The cancer continuum is the stretch of time and activities between the screening of cancer through diagnosis, treatment, remission, and possibly recurrence. Survivorship begins at the moment of cancer detection and lasts throughout the lives of those affected by cancer.

What is screening?

Screening is the process of identifying a disease or condition in individuals who show *no* signs or symptoms for the disease or condition. Screening for cancer may involve identifying a condition that may lead to cancer plus identifying the presence of cancer itself. Some types of cancer can be found before they cause symptoms. However, not all types of cancer have screening tests and some tests are only for individuals with specific genetic risks.

Screening tests for cancer may include one or more of the following:

- Medical history: a history of past illnesses and conditions with their treatment, medications, family medical history, and current symptoms (if any) will be discussed.
- Physical exam: an exam of the body with a focus on bodily systems (e.g. cardiac, lungs, neurological, muscular) will be performed.
- Laboratory tests: an examination of samples of blood and/or urine. Some laboratory tests may require a biopsy in order to evaluate the tissue under a microscope for tumor cells.
- Diagnostic Imaging: procedures such as x-ray's, computed tomography (CT) scans, magnetic resonance imaging (MRI), and sonography/ultrasound (US) may be performed.
- Genetic tests: an exam of fluid, blood, and/or tissue for DNA and RNA (ribonucleic acid) that may look for certain mutations that are linked to some types of cancer.

WHAT ARE THE GOALS OF CANCER SCREENING TESTS?

- To detect cancer before symptoms are present
- To screen for a type of cancer that is easier to treat and possibly cure when detected early
- To detect cancer without false-positive or false-negative test results
- To decrease the possibility of dying from the type of cancer that is being screened for.

It is important to note that screening tests may detect cancer but do *not*, in and of themselves, diagnose cancer. Additional testing may be necessary to diagnose a type of cancer; the process of undergoing these tests is termed 'diagnostic testing' and may include one or more of the screening tests listed above.

SHOULD EVERYONE UNDERGO CANCER SCREENING TESTS?

There are some cancer screening tests that health care professionals, scientists, and agencies/national organizations recommend in the form of guidelines for the screening of common cancers based on certain factors (e.g. age, gender, and race/ethnic groups). These cancer screening guidelines are discussed in Chapter 8.

Some individuals are at increased risk for certain cancers due to a previous history of cancer, family history of those types of cancers that may be genetic, or have exposures or risk factors that may be connected to certain types of cancer. As stated previously, having any of the previously-mentioned risks does *not* mean that individuals will develop cancer. Some screening tests are used for individuals who have known risk factors for certain types of cancer. These individuals *may* need (*not must need*) to be screened at an earlier age or at a more frequent rate than individuals without known risks for certain cancers.

Are screening tests always correct in detecting cancer?

No, screening tests are not always correct in detecting cancer although correct cancer detection is the goal of testing. False-positive and false-negative test results are possible. A 'false-positive' test shows the presence of cancer but there is not actually cancer present. A 'false-negative' test shows there is no presence of cancer but there is actually cancer present. Making the decision to undergo cancer screening tests can be difficult; learning more about the individual tests, their benefits and risks, and talking over these topics with trusted health care providers can assist in decision-making.

ARE THERE RISKS TO CANCER SCREENING TESTS?

Most screening tests have risks such as temporary discomfort, bleeding, damage to nearby tissue, or exposure to radiation. Knowing whether the screening test has been shown to decrease the possibility of dying from the cancer is important before the test is undertaken.

DOES CANCER SCREENING AT THE RECOMMENDED TIME POINT HELP EXTEND LIFE?

Scientific studies have shown that some screening tests are helpful in both detecting certain types of cancer early and in decreasing the possibility that individuals die from these types of cancer when detected early. A cancer screening test that is determined to be useful has the following attributes:

- A documented increase in the amount of cancers detected in the earlier stages.
- A documented decrease in the amount of cancers detected in the later stages.
- A documented decrease in the number of deaths related to that particular cancer.

There are other screening tests that have been shown in scientific studies to detect a certain type of cancer in some individuals before symptoms appear but the tests have not been proven to decrease the possibility that individuals die from these types of cancer. For example, if a certain type of cancer spreads quickly and is fast-growing, detecting it early through screening may not extend life.

WHAT IS THE DIFFERENCE BETWEEN A 'STANDARD' TEST AND 'POSSIBLE' TEST?

A 'standard' screening test has been found to be safe and effective for detecting the cancer such as physical exam, diagnostic imaging techniques, and tumor markers.

A 'possible' screening test may detect cancer but the test itself continues to be under study and not yet found to be safe and/or effective. More often, the 'efficacy' aspect of the possible screening test remains under study before it is viewed as a 'standard' screening test. Examples are certain diagnostic imaging techniques or one or more tumor makers. **Table 6** lists standard and possible screening tests by cancer type.

Table 6. Screening Tests by Cancer Type		
Cancer Type	*Standard Screening Test*	*Possible Screening Test (s)*
Bladder	None	Cystoscopy, Urine Cytology
Breast	Mammogram, Clinical Breast Exam, Magnetic Resonance Imaging	Thermography, Tissue Sampling
Cervical	Pap test	
Colorectal	Fecal Occult Blood test, Sigmoidoscopy, Barium enema, Colonoscopy	Virtual Colonoscopy, DNA stool test
Endometrial	None	Pap Test, Transvaginal ultrasound, Endometrial sampling
Esophageal	None	Esophagoscopy, Biopsy, Brush Cytology, Balloon cytology, Chromoendoscopy, Fluorescence spectroscopy
Stomach (Gastric)	None	Barium-meal photofluorography, upper endoscopy, serum pepsinogen
Liver	None	Ultrasound, CT scan, Tumor Markers (Alpha-fetoprotein)
Lung	Chest X-ray, Sputum cytology, low-dose spiral CT scan	
Oral cancer	None, oral exam may performed during a routine dental exam	If lesions are seen on an oral exam, tissue stains, cytology, or biopsies may be performed

Ovarian cancer	None	Pelvic exam, transvaginal ultrasound, Tumor markers (CA-125)
Prostate cancer	None	Digital rectal exam, Tumor marker [(Prostate-specific antigen (PSA)]
Skin cancer	Skin examination	If lesions are seen on a skin exam, a biopsy and/or an excision may be performed
Testicular cancer	None	Self-examination or routine physical examination

FOR WHICH CANCERS ARE SCREENING SUMMARIES AVAILABLE?

The National Cancer Institute has developed cancer screening summaries that identify and explain screening tests based on results from scientific studies about cancer risk and cancer screening tests. Versions written specifically for patients and for health care professionals are available from http://www.cancer.gov/cancertopics/pdq/screening.

Cancer screening guidelines by tumor type are discussed further in Chapter 8.

§

REFERENCES

American Cancer Society (2014), *Cancer Screening Guidelines*, http://www.cancer.org/healthy/findcancerearly/cancerscreeningguidelines/index

National Cancer Institute (2014), *Screening Testing to Detect Cancer*, http://www.cancer.gov/cancertopics/screening.

RESOURCES

American Cancer Society (2014), *Medicare Coverage for Cancer Prevention and Early Detection*, http://www.cancer.org/healthy/findcancerearly/cancerscreening-guidelines/medicare-coverage-for-cancer-prevention-and-early-detection

CANCER CONTINUUM:
DETECTION AND DIAGNOSIS

HOW IS CANCER DETECTION DIFFERENT THAN CANCER DIAGNOSIS?

The detection of cancer. is not the same as diagnosis of cancer. Cancer may be detected when symptoms or abnormalities, such as a lump or growth, are recognized by a patient or health care provider. After a cancer is detected, it still must be carefully diagnosed. A *diagnosis* is an identification of a particular type of cancer. When making a diagnosis, the initial signs and symptoms are reviewed through a variety of tests in order to see whether cancer is causing them and, if so, what *type* of cancer is causing the signs/symptoms. For example, lymphoma *may be detected* when a patient notices an enlarged lymph node, but it *must be carefully evaluated* with a number of tests in order to determine an accurate diagnosis. The diagnosis describes what type of lymphoma it is and if the cancer has metastasized.

Early detection of cancer can positively affect the outcome of the disease for *some* types of cancers. When cancer is detected, a health care provider (along with the health care team) will determine what type it is and how fast it is growing. Whether the cancer has spread nearby tissue or to other parts of the body can also be determined. In some cases, finding cancer early may decrease the risk of dying from the cancer. For this reason, improving early detection methods is a high priority for scientists and the health care team.

WHAT STEPS ARE TAKEN AFTER DETECTION?
As with screening for cancer, the detection and diagnosis phases may include one or more of the following:

- Referral to consultants to conduct:
  - o Medical history to confirm previous information and focus more on possible connections with family medical history and environmental exposures to gain further insight into the clinical picture.
  - o Physical exam to confirm previous physical findings (normal and abnormal findings) and further evaluate any original signs or symptoms of cancer (also known as *presenting* signs or symptoms)
- Laboratory tests: repeat any initial laboratory tests to confirm findings (especially if seen in a facility different than the original facility) and additional of tumor markers specific for certain cancers. Also, if tissue is obtained and a diagnosis of cancer is made, this tissue may be submitted to an outside facility for a second opinion to confirm

the original interpretation made by the pathology team.

- <u>Diagnostic Imaging</u>: additional procedures such as x-rays, CT scans, MRI, and US may be performed to determine if there is spread of the cancer beyond the original tissue site. Also, the diagnostic imaging may be submitted to an outside facility for a second opinion to confirm the original interpretation made by the radiology team.
- <u>Genetic tests</u>: additional genetic testing may be requested by consultants.

§

References

American Cancer Society (2014), *Cancer Screening Guidelines*, http://www.cancer.org/healthy/findcancerearly/cancerscreeningguidelines/index

National Cancer Institute (2014), *Screening Testing to Detect Cancer*, http://www.cancer.gov/cancertopics/screening

CANCER CONTINUUM: TREATMENT

HOW IS CANCER TREATED?

The treatment of cancer is a delicate balance of preference, goals, knowledge, timing, access to care (including clinical trials), availability, finances, and joint decision-making between the patient-family-caregiver-health care provider team.

Treatment methods of cancer may include one or more of the following conventional approaches listed in **Table 7**. Some of these categories overlap one another, and some cancer treatment regimens may use one or more of these approaches.

Table 7. Cancer Treatment Methods: Definitions and Examples		
Treatment Method	*Definition*	*Example(s)*
Surgery	An operation to remove or repair a part of the body or to find out if disease is present	Biopsy, Lumpectomy, Resection
Radiation Therapy	The use of high-energy radiation from x-rays, gamma rays, neutrons, protons, and other sources to kill cancer cells and shrink tumors.	External beam radiation, Brachytherapy
Chemotherapy	Treatment with drugs given orally, topically, intravenously, intra-arterial, and/or intra-peritoneal that kill cancer cells by stopping or slowing the growth of cells	Paclitaxel, Doxorubicin, Cyclophosphamide

Targeted Therapies	A type of treatment that uses drugs or other substances to identify and attack specific types of cancer cells by blocking the action of certain enzymes, proteins, or other molecules involved in the growth and spread of cancer cells. Other types of targeted therapies help the immune system kill cancer cells or deliver toxic substances directly to cancer cells and kill them.	Monoclonal antibodies, Vascular endothelial growth factor, Cytokines, Immunomodulaters

Transplantation	A procedure in which tissue, blood, or an organ is transferred from one area of a person's body to another area, or from one person (the donor) to another person (the recipient).	Liver transplant, Kidney transplant, Bone marrow transplant, Peripheral blood stem cell transplant
Biological Therapies	Treatment that uses substances made from living organisms to treat disease. Some therapies stimulate or suppress the immune system; Other therapies attack specific cancer cells.	Immunotherapy (such as vaccines, cytokines, and some antibodies), gene therapy, and some targeted therapies, Biological response modifier therapy
Vaccine Therapy	Treatment that uses a substance to stimulate the immune system to destroy a tumor or infectious bacteria or viruses.	Prostate cancer vaccine
Cryotherapy	Any method that uses cold temperature to treat disease	Cryoablation for prostate cancer

Hyperthermia Therapy	Treatment in which body tissue is open to higher temperatures to destroy and kill cancer cells or to make cancer cells more sensitive to the impact of radiation and certain anticancer drugs	Local hyperthermia, Thermal ablation
Laser Therapy	Treatment that uses strong beams of light to cut and destroy tissue. Laser	Transpupillary thermotherapy for eye melanoma; Laser therapy for lymphedema after
	therapy may also be used to reduce swelling caused by a buildup of lymph fluid in tissue	breast cancer surgery
Photodynamic Therapy	Treatment with drugs that become active when exposed to light. These activated drugs may kill cancer cells.	Phototherapy, portimer sodium used as a photosensitizer in the treatment of cancer of the esophagus or non-small cell lung cancer

WHAT IS 'WATCHFUL WAITING' AND 'ACTIVE SURVEILLANCE?'

'Watchful waiting' and 'active surveillance' are types of expectant medical management. Watchful waiting is thoroughly and closely observing a patient's condition but not treating unless symptoms appear or the symptoms change in nature. Watchful waiting is sometimes used in prostate cancer management and can be used in any situation where the medical condition progresses slowly or when the risks of treatment are greater than the likely benefits. During the thorough and close observation period, certain exams and tests are performed on a regular schedule.

'Active surveillance' is a treatment plan that also thoroughly and closely observes a patient's condition but not giving any treatment unless there are changes in test results that show the condition is getting worse. Active surveillance may be used in the treatment of certain types of cancer, such as urethral cancer and intraocular (eye) melanoma. Active surveillance may be used to avoid or postpone the need for treatment such as radiation therapy or surgery. As with watchful waiting, during active surveillance, certain exams and tests are performed on a regular schedule.

Cancer treatment guidelines by tumor type is discussed further in Chapter 9.

Cancer Continuum: Remission and Disease-Free Survival

What is the difference between remission and disease-free status?

'Remission' is a decrease in or disappearance of signs and symptoms of cancer. A *partial* remission is the disappearance of some, but not all, signs and symptoms of cancer. A *complete* remission is the disappearance of all signs and symptoms of cancer although cancer still may be present in the body but not visible on diagnostic imaging.

'Disease-free' survival is the length of time after the treatment (usually primary treatment) ends and before new signs and symptoms of the original cancer appear again. Cancer cannot be detected during a disease-free status.

Cancer can be a long-term, chronic illness in the absence of a remission or a disease-free survival time period. Cancer may respond to treatment in what is known as a *partial response* in that the disease partially responded to treatment but did not completely disappear. Often, a partial response is a decrease in half of the original amount of the tumor or 50% reduction in the tumor's measurement. Researchers suggest that the reduction in the size of the tumor must be sustained for a minimum of one month to be considered in 'response' status.

Cancer Continuum: Progression and Recurrence

What is the difference between progression and recurrence?

'Progression' of disease is when a tumor grows larger or metastasizes after being in a 'stable' disease state (not growing or spreading). Disease 'progression' during or soon after treatment may prompt an extension or change in the treatment plan.

'Recurrence' is the return of the cancer usually following a period of disease-free status to the primary or original site or to another place in the body. In either situation, the primary tumor type remains the same.

If recurrence occurs, does it mean that the original cancer wasn't treated completely?

When recurrence happens, an evaluation of the tumor's location and any new signs or symptoms will be performed. Since not all cancer types are treated in the same manner, treatment of recurrent cancer requires consideration of several aspects, not limited to the following: (a) type or cancer, (b) location of the cancer, (c) extent of disease and areas of metastasis [if present], (d) tolerance of the previous treatment regimen, (e) current health status, (f) availability/efficacy/safety of new treatment regimens, and (g) patient preferences.

Cancer Continuum: End of Life Care

What are the goals of end of life care?

When the decision is made to no longer provide primary treatment for the underlying disease(s)/condition(s), medical and nursing care is *active* and focused on noticing and treating symptoms. Common symptoms for which medications are available to treat are pain, restlessness, nausea, constipation, and difficulty breathing. Some of the following symptoms often signal that the end of life is near: drowsiness, confusion, decreased socialization, loss of appetite, cool skin, loss of bladder or bowel control. See Chapter 3 for more information on cancer-related symptoms.

Are there resources available for family and friends and caregivers?

Resources for family, friends, and caregivers are plentiful and growing. More effort has been dedicated in the past few decades to assisting individuals who are caring for and supporting those with cancer facing the end of life. Booklets can be printed on demand or ordered in bulk on many helpful topics include these:

- "When Someone You Love Has Advanced Cancer: Support for Caregivers" http://www.cancer.gov/cancertopics/coping/when-someone-you-love-has-advanced-cancer
- "Facing Forward: When Some You Love Has Completed Cancer Treatment" http://www.cancer.gov/cancertopics/coping/someone-you-love-completed-cancer-treatment
- Nearing the End of Life http://www.cancer.org/treatment/nearingtheendoflife/nearingtheendoflife/nearing-the-end-of-life-toc
- Choosing Home Care http://www.cancer.org/treatment/nearingtheendoflife/nearingtheendoflife/nearing-the-end-of-life-home-care
- Choosing Hospice Care http://www.cancer.org/treatment/nearingtheendoflife/nearingtheendoflife/nearing-the-end-of-life-hospice

3

Cancer Symptom Management

How is symptom management important in cancer care?

Symptom management is the recognition, evaluation, and ongoing interventions necessary to relieve signs and symptoms associated with the disease process and/or its treatment. The management of symptoms is as important in cancer care as treatment for the cancer itself. Untreated or less-than-optimally treated symptoms may impact patient outcomes and/or contribute to an overall difficult patient experience (Lee, 2010, handbook p. 69). Often, when symptoms are recognized, properly and fully evaluated, and a treatment plan is in place, patients can better tolerate the treatment for the disease itself. Treatment plans are generally made jointly between patient, caregiver, and healthcare team.

WHAT ARE SOME OF THE CANCER-RELATED SYMPTOMS THAT REQUIRE A TREATMENT PLAN?

Any symptom that is distressing, in other words, causes discomfort or inhibits quality of life, may be treated if this is the patient's preference. Often, symptoms occur at the same time with other symptoms and this phenomenon is called 'symptom clusters'. A common example is the occurrence of pain, fatigue, and sleep pattern changes at the same time, each adding negatively to the whole experience. A list of possible signs and symptoms with a brief description are seen in **Table 8**.

Table 8. Possible Signs and Symptoms in Cancer Care

Signs and Symptoms	Brief Descriptions
Alopecia	Hair loss
Altered body image and sexual health	Changes in self-worth due to physical appearance or feelings
Anemia	Decreased hemoglobin
Anorexia-Cachexia Syndrome	Loss of appetite or desire to eat
Anxiety	Feelings of tension or worry
Arthralgias and myalgias	Joint or muscle aches
Bladder disturbances	Increased or painful urination
Bleeding and thrombotic complications	Uncontrolled or spontaneous bleeding
Cerebellar syndromes	Changes in walking and balance
Cognitive dysfunction	Changes in ability to process thoughts or remember topics
Constipation	Slowed bowel function
Depression	Persistent change in the way one thinks about life
Diarrhea	Increased bowel function
Dysphagia	Difficulty swallowing
Dyspnea	Difficulty breathing
Effusions	Fluid collection in body areas not supposed to collect fluid (e.g. heart, lungs)
Electrolyte imbalances	Changes in normal levels of some elements such as sodium or potassium in the blood
Fatigue	Persistent tiredness or exhaustion
Flu-like symptoms	Fever, body aches, chills, fatigue
Increased intracranial pressure	Serious changes in the pressure in the brain restricting blood flow
Infection	Invasion of the body by disease-causing microorganisms
Loss and Grief	Sadness and mourning following perhaps a loss of one's health
Lymphedema	Fluid collection in the lymph-areas of the body (e.g. arms, legs)

Malignant Ascites	Fluid collection in body areas not supposed to collect fluid (e.g. lining of the abdomen)
Menopausal symptoms	Hot flashes, emotional changes, headaches, insomnia
Mucositis	Inflamed lining of the mouth
Myelosuppression	Marked decrease in the amount of functioning cells in the bone marrow and blood stream
Nausea and vomiting	Queasy sensation with
Neutropenia	Serious decrease of functioning white blood cells
Pain	Discomfort that may be mild,
	moderate, or severe
Peripheral Neuropathy	Numbness and tingling in arms and/or legs
Pruritis	Itching
Skin and nail bed changes	Dryness, cracking, discoloration
Skin ulcerations	Sores of varying depths and location
Sleep Disturbances	Difficulty falling asleep or remaining asleep
Spinal Cord Compression	Pressure on the spinal cord by bone, tumor, or an abscess
Spiritual Distress	Changes in personal spirituality framework including outlook and hopefulness
Taste Changes	Inability to taste or unpleasant changes in normal tasting
Thrombocytopenia	Serious decrease of functioning platelets which help with clotting
Xerostomia	Severe and uncomfortable dry mouth

§

References

Brown, C (2010) *A Guide to Oncology Symptom Management.* Pittsburgh: Oncology Nursing Society Publishing Division.

Lee, C. & Decker, G. (2012). *Cancer and Complementary Medicine: Your Guide to Smart Choices in Symptom Management.* Pittsburgh: Oncology Nursing Society Publishing Division.

National Cancer Institute, *NCI Dictionary of Cancer Terms,* http://www.cancer.gov/dictionary

4

INTEGRATIVE ONCOLOGY:
COMPLEMENTARY AND
ALTERNATIVE MEDICINE

To this point, the discussion has centered on conventional cancer care, that is, therapies that are part of the standard of care with profiles of efficacy and safety for cancer treatment. Typically, conventional care is also termed 'western' or 'allopathic' or 'traditional' medicine.

WHAT IS COMPLEMENTARY AND ALTERNATIVE MEDICINE?

Complementary and/or alternative medicine (CAM) is traditional medicine combined with CAM approaches (complementary) or instead of (alternative) traditional approaches. Medical interventions relying on natural healing

(19th century term), drugless healing (early 20th century term), or holistic healing (1970s to present term) are not new or original in the US as the history of CAM dates back to the 1700s. Terms used today in CAM are listed in **Table 9**.

The use of CAM and surveys measuring its use has been increasing steadily in recent decades. Data from the 2007 National Center for Health Statistics (NCHS)/NCCAM survey indicated that 38% of US adults had used some form of CAM therapy during the previous 12 months (Barnes, Bloom, & Nahin, 2008). This survey compared results to the 2002 published survey (Barnes, Powell-Griner, McFann, & Nahin, 2004).

Table 9. Complementary and Alternative Medicine Terms	
Term	*Definition*
Complementary medicine	Traditional medicine that is combine with CAM approaches.
Alternative medicine	Traditional medicine that is used instead of traditional approaches.
Integrative medicine	Traditional medicine combined with evidence-based complementary therapies; Focuses on health promotion versus disease prevention and access to lower-cost, evidence-based therapies.
Integrative oncology	Integrative medicine combined with evidence-based oncology care; Focuses on a comprehensive health approach to the human body, mind, soul, and spirit.

HOW DID NATIONAL INTEREST IN CAM BEGIN?

Public education, legislative action, and medical advances in the mid-1970s to 1980s did not deter US patients from seeking CAM. To address the growing and important issues, the Office of Alternative Medicine (OAM) was established in 1992, becoming the National Center for Complementary and Alternative Medicine in 1998. NCCAM is one of the 27 institutes and centers that make up the National Institutes of Health (NIH), which is one of eight agencies under the Public Health Service (PHS) in the U.S. Department of Health and Human Services (DHHS). NCCAM conducts and funds CAM research across many diseases and conditions and serves as a repository for educational materials for healthcare providers, patients, and the community.

To increase the amount of high-quality information and research CAM use, the NIH established the Office of Cancer Complementary and Alternative Medicine within the National Cancer Institute (NCI) in 1998. The OCCAM sponsors research within CAM disciplines and therapies as they relate to the prevention, diagnosis, and treatment of cancer, cancer-related symptoms, and side effects of conventional treatment. OCCAM maintains a current listing of clinical trials involving CAM therapies for the treatment of cancer and cancer-related symptoms in addition to all cancer CAM clinical trials no longer enrolling participants (closed) (http://cam.cancer.gov/clinicaltrials_table.html).

Cancer CAM clinical trials are currently tracked for the following cancers:

- Adrenocortical
- Bladder
- Breast
- Colon
- Endometrial
- Esophageal
- Head and neck
- Leukemia
- Lung cancer (small cell/non-small cell)
- Lymphoma
- Melanoma
- Mesothelioma
- Neuroendocrine skin cancer
- Pancreatic
- Prostate
- Rectal

Cancer CAM clinical trials are currently tracked for the following symptoms:

- Anorexia
- Hot flashes
- Fatigue
- Nausea

- Oral complications
- Pain

WHAT IS THE WHITE HOUSE COMMISSION ON CAM POLICY?

The White House Commission on Complementary and Alternative Medicine Policy (WHCCAMP) was established in March 2000 to address issues of access to and delivery of CAM, priorities for research, and the need to educate consumers and health professionals. The outcome was the development of guiding principles. A non-government agency established in 1970, the Institute of Medicine (IOM) of the National Academies sponsored meetings in 2003-2004 to explore scientific, policy, and practice questions that arise from the increasing use of CAM use in the US. The outcome was the development of model guidelines. The final report of the IOM committee was released in January 2005. Ultimately, the WHCC guiding principles and IOM model guidelines remain the only existing framework for CAM utilization on a national level and have not been revised in over a decade.

HOW DID ACADEMIC INTEREST IN CAM BEGIN?

The Consortium of Academic Health Centers for Integrative Medicine (CAHCIM), first established in

2004, has grown to include 56 academic medical centers and affiliate institutions in the US and Canada. CAHCIM's mission is to advance academic centers' principles and practices of integrative medicine through education, research, and policy development. In 2010, the NCI OCCAM and NCI's Office of Communications and Education conducted an inventory of integrative medicine programs (IMP) in NCI Cancer Centers and other academic institution-based health centers across the country. Sixty-six NCI cancer centers and 41 IMPs participated. While the inventory showed that additional inquiry is needed, collaborating activities involving cancer care and CAM modalities between CCPs and IMPs are ongoing (Mikhail, et al, 2012). These collaborations demonstrate an interest to broaden traditional cancer care to include evidence-based complementary therapies, relevant education, and the development of high-quality research.

WHICH PROFESSIONAL SOCIETIES HAVE AN INTEREST IN CAM?

The professional association solely dedicated to the integration of CAM practice, education, and research into cancer care is the Society for Integrative Oncology (SIO). A non-profit organization founded in 2003, SIO's mission is to promote evidence-based integrative care to improve the lives of those impacted by cancer. SIO published its first iteration of evidence-based, clinical *Practice Guidelines for Integrative Oncology* in 2007 which were later amended and made public in 2009 (Deng et al., 2009). The guidelines are for clinicians to use when making clinical choices for their patients. Additionally, the guidelines may be a source document for quality assurance and multidisciplinary care.

§

REFERENCES

Barnes, P.M., Bloom, B., & Nahin, R.L. (2008). *Complementary and alternative medicine use among adults and children: United States*, 2007. National Health Statistics Reports, 12, 1-23.

Barnes, P. M., Powell-Griner, E., McFann, K., & Nahin, R. L. (2004). Complementary and alternative medicine use among adults: United States, 2002. Adv Data(343), 1-19.

Committee on the Use of Complementary and Alternative Medicine by the American Public, Institute of Medicine of the National Academies. (2005). Complementary and alternative medicine in the United States. Washington, DC: National Academies Press

Consortium of Academic Health Centers for Integrative Medicine. (2013). Consortium of Academic Health Centers for Integrative Medicine. Retrieved August 17, 2013, from http://www.imconsortium.org/about/home.html

Deng, G.E., Frenkel, M., Cohen, L., Cassileth, B.R., Abrams, D.I., Capodice, J.L., Courneya, K.Sa., Dryden, T., Hanser, S., Kumar, N., Labriola, D., Wardell, D.W., Sagar, S. (2009). Evidence-based clinical practice guidelines for integrative oncology: complementary therapies and botanicals. Journal of the Society for Integrative Oncology, *7*(3), 85-120.

Mikhail I, Austin, E., Buckman, S, Lee, C., Goodman, N., White, J.: P03.14. Cancer complementary and alternative medicine research among NCI's cancer centers program and the integrative medicine programs: an inventory. BMC Complementary and Alternative Medicine 2012 12(Suppl 1):P267 doi:10.1186/1472-6882-12-S1-P267

Mumber, M.P. (2006). Principles of integrative oncology. In M.P. Mumber (Ed.), *Integrative oncology principles and practice* (pp. 3–15). New York: Taylor and Francis.

National Center for Complementary and Alternative Medicine. (2013a). *Complementary, Alternative, or Integrative Health: What's In a Name?* Retrieved August 4, 2013, from http://nccam.nih.gov/health/whatiscam.

Society for Integrative Oncology. (2013). SIO Mission. Retrieved August 17, 2013 from http://www.integrativeonc. org/

U.S. Department of Health and Human Services. (2002). *White House Commission on Complementary and Alternative Medicine Policy* [NIH Publication No. 03-5411]. Washington, DC: U.S. Government Printing Office.

Resources

Cohen, L. & Markman, M. (Eds.) (2008). *Integrative Oncology. Incorporating Complementary Medicine into Conventional Cancer Care.* New Jersey: Humana Press.

Cohen, M., Ruggie, M., & Micozzi, M.S. (2007). *The Practice of Integrative Medicine: A Legal and Operational Guide.* New York: Springer Publishing Company.

Mumber, M.P. (Ed). (2006). *Integrative Oncology: Principles and Practice.* London: Taylor & Francis

Decker, G.M. (Ed). (1999). *An Introduction to Complementary & Alternative Therapies.* Pittsburgh: Oncology Nursing Press, Inc.

American Cancer Society Complete Guide to Complementary & Alternative Cancer Therapies (2009, 2nd Edition), Georgia: American Cancer Society.

Alternative Medicine: Your Guide to Stress Relief, Healing, Nutrition, and More. TIME (2012). New York: Time Books.

5

THE CANCER CARE TEAM

WHO ARE THE MEMBERS OF THE CANCER TEAM?

Cancer care teams are composed of an array of health care providers, specialists, and support person dedicated to the care of the individual with cancer and his/her support network. Oftentimes, these teams are 'multidisciplinary' composed of health care professional across multiple disciplines. Who coordinates the team depends on the type of cancer, its stage, and where the care is sought. Most often, a team composed of a physician and non-physician providers serve as the core group, such as an oncologist with either a nurse practitioner or physician assistant, and an oncology nurse. The three main types of oncologists are medical, surgical, and radiation oncologists. Examples of other subspecialty types of oncologists are age-based oncologists [pediatric, geriatric] and organ-based oncologists [gynecologic, hematology]. **Table 10** lists types of oncologists and other specialized physicians and the focus of their care.

Table 10. Physician in Cancer Care and Focus of Care	
Physician Type	*Primary Focus of Care*
Diagnostic Radiologist	Diagnoses disease using imaging tests such as mammograms, ultrasounds, X-rays, MRI, CT, and PET scans*
Gastroenterologist	Specializes in the diagnosis and treatment of digestive system cancers*
Geriatric Oncologist	Specializes in the medical treatment of older adults with cancer *
Gynecologic oncologist	Specializes in the diagnosis, care and treatment of gynecologic cancers such as uterine, cervical, or ovarian cancer*
Hematologist-Oncologist	Specializes in the diagnosis and treatment of blood disorders including cancers of the blood such as leukemia, lymphoma, and multiple myeloma*
Hospice and Palliative Care Physicians	Specialize in the prevention and relief of suffering throughout the care continuum*
Medical Oncologist	Specializes in care from the time of diagnosis throughout the course of the disease*
Neurosurgeon	Specializes in brain, spinal cord, or nerve-related operations*

Pulmonologist	Specializes in the diagnosis and treatment of respiratory tract cancers*
Radiation Oncologist	Specializes in treating cancer with radiation therapy*
Surgical Oncologist	Specializes in the surgical management of cancer (removal of the tumor and surrounding tissue during an operation or biopsy)*
Pediatric Oncologist	Specializes in the treatment of children with cancer*
Specialty Referrals/Consults	Referrals geared toward addressing new or recurring problems during care including: Pain, Neurology, Dental, Psychiatric, Infectious Disease, and Podiatry, among others*

* Possesses advanced training through residency and fellowship programs; may be board certified

In addition to oncologists, an array of health care providers/professionals (HCPs) contribute to the team at one time or another in the course of the cancer care spectrum. **Table 11** lists these some of these HCPs and the focus of their care.

Table 11. Health Care Professionals in Cancer Care and Focus of Care	
Health Care Professional	**Primary Focus of Care**
Advanced Practice Nurse (APRNs)	Nurses with masters, doctorates of nursing practice, or PhDs in nursing who work with a high level of independence
Cancer Case Manager*	Coordinates care throughout the cancer care spectrum
Cancer Registrars	Specialize in the collection and analysis of regional and national cancer research data
Dietitian*	Monitors nutritional status in an inpatient or outpatient setting, recommends and educates regarding food choices
Home health nurse*	Specializes in providing nursing care in the home including medications, dressing changes, teaching about self-care
Genetic Counselors*	Specializes in education about genetic test results and helps with informed decision-making with the health care team
Nurse Practitioner*	Specializes in the diagnoses and management of illness; can order medications including chemotherapy in some states; an Advanced Practice Nurse
Occupational Therapist*	Specializes in assisting individuals with re-learning activities of daily living
Oncology Nurse (Clinic, Hospital, Rural)*	Specializes in the care of cancer patients; may administer chemotherapy, blood products, assist with

	procedures, coordinate care among the cancer care team.
Oncology Clinical Nurse Specialist*	Specializes in the care of cancer patients; may provide direct care, supervise staff, conduct research, and/or teach patients, staff, families about cancer care; an Advanced Practice Nurse
Oncology Clinical Pharmacists*	Specialize in the dispensing of anticancer therapies and medications to reduce side effects of treatment
Oncology Nurse Practitioner*	Specializes in care from the time of diagnosis throughout the course of the disease; has advanced training and clinical experience; can order medications including chemotherapy in some states.; an Advanced Practice Nurse
Oncology Social Worker*	Specializes in counseling, advocacy and referrals for financial, spiritual and behavioral health needs
Patient Navigator*	Specialize in guiding patients and families through the treatment process through survivorship phase
Physical Therapist*	Specializes in the examination, testing, and treatment of individuals to restore or maintain strength, function, and/or mobility

Physician Assistant*	Specializes in the diagnoses and management of illness; can order medications including chemotherapy in some states.; works alongside physicians
Respiratory Therapist*	Specializes in providing breathing treatments and education on self-administration

*May possess bachelors and masters degrees in area of specialty and board certification
** Possesses advanced training through residency and fellowship programs; may be board certification

6

Guidelines and the Standard of Care: An Introduction

What have we covered so far?

To this point, we have covered the foundational components of cancer care: how it begins, how it is detected, diagnosed and treated; the importance of symptom management and the emerging face of integrative oncology. Before we can address how best to approach cancer care, we need to develop a solid understanding of how health care decision-making occurs and the reference platforms that provide the basis for these decisions in the medical and nursing arenas.

HOW DO HEALTH CARE PROVIDERS MAKE CLINICAL DECISIONS?

Healthcare providers are often faced with challenging choices and uncertainty when treating patients. Providers rely on scientific literature, their knowledge, skills, experience, and patient preferences to inform their decision-making. Pre-established healthcare standards and clinical practice guidelines assist not only the provider but patients and family members as well in navigating the sometimes challenging choices that accompany healthcare. Every patient desires to receive care that has been universally accepted by experts as the proper treatment, otherwise known as the standard of care. Understanding what each of these concepts mean (standards, guidelines, standard of care) and how they intersect is important in understanding what is at stake when the standard of care is not met.

WHAT ARE HEALTH CARE STANDARDS?

Health care standards are criteria that are relied upon to guide decision-making in clinical care. Decision-making involves choosing the best treatment, valuing outcomes, interpreting diagnostic information, deciding when and how to test, finding the evidence summarizing the evidence, and, finally, making the decision (s).

Decision-making in medical and nursing care should be based upon evidence-based information gained from experts, peer-reviewed resources, and relevant clinical experience. Most often, standards and guidelines are relied upon to form a foundational framework by which health care providers can combine with literature findings, consultation with peers, and clinical experience. This multi-stage framework approach forms the standard of care.

WHAT IS 'STANDARD OF CARE'?

Standard of care is treatment that is accepted by experts as a proper treatment for a certain type of disease or condition that is widely used by healthcare professionals. It is also defined as the degree of skill and judgment by a prudent health provider under similar circumstances Standards of care are also called best practice, standard medical care, standard therapy or standard operating procedure.

WHAT ARE 'GUIDELINES'?

Guidelines are summary statements that identify and evaluate high quality evidence about the prevention, diagnosis, prognosis, risk/benefit considerations, and cost-effectiveness of treatment plans. They define important questions and identify possible decision options and their outcomes. Some guidelines contain decision-making 'trees' or algorithms to guide the next steps in diagnosis and/or treatment plans. Guidelines are used to standardize care, raise the quality of care, and reduce risk (whether it be to the patient, provider, insurer) with a focus on safe, effective, and cost-conscious care.

WHAT ARE CLINICAL PRACTICE GUIDELINES?

One of the most common type of guidelines are clinical practice guidelines (CPGs). CPGs are statements developed to assist in decision-making about the screening, prevention, or treatment of specific clinical conditions. CPGs are also known as best practice, clinical guidelines, medical guidelines, or clinical protocols. The intent of CPGs is to optimize health care. CPGs are informed by a systematic review (SR) of evidence and an assessment of the benefits and harms of the alternative health options.

WHAT IS EVIDENCE-BASED HEALTH CARE?

Evidence-based health care is the use of current best evidence in making decisions about the care of patients or the delivery of health services. Current best evidence is up-to-date information from relevant, valid research about the effects of various forms of health care, possible harm from certain exposures, accuracy of diagnostic testing, and strength of predictions regarding prognosis for a condition.

What is evidence-based clinical practice?

Evidence-based clinical practice is an approach to decision-making in which the health care provider/team uses the best available evidence to decide upon the option which suits that patient best in collaboration *with* the patient. It is also referred to a evidence-based practice

What is evidence-based medicine?

Evidence-based medicine (EBM) is the use of current best evidence in making decisions about the medical care of patients. Practicing EBM means integrating individual clinical expertise with the best available research evidence. Essentially, EBM is the connection between individual clinical expertise, best external evidence, and patient values, preference, and expectations.

Table 12 summarizes various terms regarding guidelines and standard of care.

Table 12. Terms & Definitions: Guidelines & Standard of Care	
Term	**Definition**
Health care standards	Criteria that guides decision – making in clinical care
Standard of Care	Widely-accepted proper treatment for a condition
Guidelines	Summary statements the identify and evaluate quality evidence
Guideline Syntheses	Comparisons of selected guidelines by topic
Clinical Practice Guidelines (CPG)	Statements informed by systematic review of evidence and assessment of benefits/harms of alternative options, also known as "best practice"
Evidence-based health care	Care based on current best evidence
Evidence-based clinical practice	Care focused on inclusion of the patient in decision-making
Evidence-based medicine (EBM)	Care focused on inclusion of clinical expertise with current best evidence
Clinical pathways	Tools, such as a clinical map, to guide evidence-based healthcare
Systematic Reviews (SR)	Synthesis of all relevant studies by topic with a detailed search strategy, many include a meta-analysis
Meta-analyses (MA)	A pooled analysis of comparable data from different research studies

§

References

Cochrane Collaboration. http://www.cochrane.org/about-us/evidence-based-health-care

Florida State University College of Medicine. Definition of Evidence-based Medicine http://med.fsu.edu/index.cfm?page=medicalinformatics.ebmTutorial

National Cancer Institute Online glossary: http://www.cancer.gov/dictionary#

CANCER-RELATED GUIDELINES AND THE STANDARD OF CARE: EXPANDED

WHO DEVELOPS GUIDELINES?

Guidelines are usually developed at the national or international level by government bodies, medical and/or, nursing professional associations. Academic programs and some large medical centers are other common guideline developers. Local healthcare providers (e.g. clinics, hospitals) may adapt guidelines from existing guidelines or develop their own. When guidelines are adapted for local use, referencing the original guideline offers credibility.

HOW IS THE US INSTITUTE OF MEDICINE INVOLVED IN CPGS?

The Institute of Medicine (IOM) is the health arm of the National Academy of Sciences (NAS) dedicated to asking and answering 'hot topics' in health and health care. After its original work in the early 1990s and after the *Medicare Improvements for Patients and Providers of 2008* was passed, the IOM developed standards for systematic reviews (SRs) for CPGs and comparative effectiveness research. The premise was that, if standards were available for developing valid SRs and CPGs, then the public and clinicians should have greater trust in these CPGs (xii, preface).

Theoretically, trustworthy CPGs could be translated into electronic formats for wide dissemination to support clinical decision-making.

Since the IOM's original work over two decades ago, specialty societies, disease advocacy groups, the federally supported U.S. Preventive Services Task Forces (USPSTF), health insurance plans, and other interested groups have developed and published guidelines totaling nearly thousands in number. At present, there are national guidelines and international guidelines that serve as resource platforms to guide clinical decision making.

To be trustworthy CPGs, according to the IOM, should (pp. 25-26):

- Be based on a SR of the evidence to date
- Be developed by a knowledgeable panel of experts
- Be based on a transparent process minimizing bias and any conflicts of interest
- Reflect patient subgroups and patient preferences
- Explain a clear relationship between the alternative care options (what 'else is out there') and health outcomes
- Provide ratings of both the quality of evidence and strength of the recommendations
- Be recognized and revised when important new evidence merits changes in the recommendations

Eight major standards for developing trustworthy clinical practice guidelines are listed in **Table 13**. The processes involved in ensuring each of these standards is completely met is outlined in the full report.

Table 13. Standards for Developing Trustworthy Clinical Practice Guidelines	
Standard	Focus Area
1	Establishing transparency
2	Management of conflict of interest
3	Guidelines development group composition
4	Clinical practice guidelines-systematic review intersection
5	Establishing evidence foundations for and rating strength of recommendations
6	Articulation of recommendations
7	External review
8	Updating

Which rating systems assessing strength of recommendations are used?

Multiple rating systems are available to systematically 'grade' the available research on a particular clinical topic. U.S. approaches cited in the *Clinical Practice Guidelines We Can Trust* are:

- Institute for Clinical Systems Improvement (2003)
- Strength of Recommendation Taxonomy (2004)
- US Preventative Services Task Force (2008)
- American College of Cardiology Foundation/ American Heart Association (2009)
- American Academy of Pediatrics (2004)
- American Academy of Neurology (2004)
- American College of Chest Physicians (2009)

- National Comprehensive Cancer Network (2008)
- Infectious Diseases Society of America (2001)

The full report is available: Standards for Developing Trustworthy Clinical Practice Guidelines [(Institute of Medicine of the National Academies) http://www.iom.edu/Reports/2011/Clinical-Practice-Guidelines-We-Can-Trust/Standards.aspx]

Guidelines and the Standard of Care Development: National Guidelines and the Guideline Clearinghouse

Where are our National Guidelines housed?

In the US, the National Guideline Clearinghouse (NGC) serves as the public source in cataloguing CPGs. The NGC is housed within the Agency for Healthcare Research and Quality [(AHRQ) in the US Department of Health and Human Services]. These guidelines are catalogued by topic area, name of the organization who developed the guideline(s) from A-Z, and those guidelines which are currently under development.

Special features of the NGC are:

- Ability to personalize specific guideline interests
- Ability to receive alerts on new and updated content
- Ability to compare guidelines by generating side-by-side comparison
- Ability to generate a table of all the guidelines at the intersection of two major fields: (a) clinical specialty and (b) methods used to analyze the evidence.

- Ability to conduct an advanced search by the following criteria: (a) target age, (b) clinical specialty, (c) guideline category, (d) intended users, (e) IOM domain, (f) methods used to analyze the evidence, (g) methods used to assess the quality and strength of the evidence, (h) publication year, (i) organizations, (j) organization type, (k) target sex of population, among others.

WHICH CLINICAL SPECIALTIES ARE REPRESENTED IN THE NGC CPGS?

Allergy & Immunology
Anesthesiology
Cardiology
Chiropractic
Colon & Rectal Surgery
Critical Care
Dentistry
Dermatology
Emergency Medicine
Endocrinology
Family Practice
Gastroenterology
Geriatrics
Hematology
Infectious Disease
Internal Medicine
Medical Genetics
Nephrology
Neurological Surgery
Neurology
Nuclear Medicine
Nursing
Nutrition
Obstetrics/Gynecology

Oncology
Ophthalmology
Optometry
Orthopedic Surgery
Otolaryngology
Pathology
Pediatrics
Pharmacology
Physical Medicine and Rehabilitation
Plastic Surgery
Podiatry
Preventive Medicine
Psychiatry
Psychology
Pulmonary Medicine
Radiation Oncology
Radiology
Rheumatology
Sleep Medicine
Speech-Language Pathology
Sports Medicine
Surgery
Thoracic Surgery
Urology

What methods are used to analyze the evidence and the quality/ strength of evidence in the Cpgs?

Meta-analyses and systematic reviews of individual patient data and trial data (e.g. observational, randomized controlled trials). The quality and strength is measured through weighting of the data according to a pre-specific rating scheme and expert consensus techniques (e.g. nominal group technique, Delphi method).

What is the Guideline Matrix and how can it locate applicable Cpgs?

The Guideline Matrix (available to the public on the website) generates a table of all the guidelines that intersection a clinical specialty and the technique used to analyze the available evidence. For example, a matrix generated for "Oncology" as the clinical specialty and "Meta-analysis of Randomized Controlled Trials" reveals 21 CPGs housed in the NPC. Of the 21 CPGs, here are some options to select from:

- Risk reduction of prostate cancer with drugs or nutritional supplements. 2012 May 17. NGC:009863
- Systemic therapy for advanced gastric cancer. 2010 Dec 16. NGC:008091
- Neuropathic pain. The pharmacological management of neuropathic pain in adults in

non-specialist settings. 2010 Mar. [NGC Update Pending] NGC:008059

- Screening for breast cancer: U.S. Preventive Services Task Force recommendation statement. 2) December 2009 addendum. 1996 (revised 2009 Nov; addendum released 2009 Dec). NGC:007533

(http://www.guideline.gov/matrix.aspx) Please see the complete report available on the public website.

GUIDELINES AND THE STANDARD OF CARE: THE JOINT COMMISSION

WHO IS THE JOINT COMMISSION?

The Joint Commission is a nationally-recognized, independent organization that accredits and certifies more than 20,000 health care programs. Founded in 1951, The Joint Commission is the nation's largest and oldest health care body that both sets standards and accredits. **Table 14** lists the types of program and examples.

Table 14. Examples of Health care Services Accredited by The Joint Commission	
Program Type	*Examples*
Ambulatory Health Care	Surgical, medical/dental, diagnostic/therapeutic services, and episodic care
Behavioral Health Care	Mental health and chemical dependency services
Critical Access Hospital Care	Selected hospitals with 25 or less beds keeping patients 96 or less hours
Home Care	Home health, personal care and/or support, home medical equipment, hospice, and pharmacy
Hospital Care	General, children's, long term acute, psychiatric, rehabilitation and specialty hospitals
Laboratory Services	Reference labs and in vitro fertilization labs, and those

	connected with hospitals and ambulatory surgical centers
Nursing Care Centers	Rehabilitation, post-acute care
Office-Based Surgery	Surgical practices with four or fewer practitioners

What are the benefits of Joint Commission accreditation?

The Joint Commission cites many benefits to accreditation, among them are:

- Strengthens patient safety efforts
- Strengthens confidence in the quality and safety of care, treatment, and services
- May serve as a recognition tool by insurers and third party payers
- May reduce liability insurance costs

In which areas does Joint Commission offer certification?

The Joint Commission offers certification opportunities for groups meeting clinically-specific evaluation requirements in the following areas:

- Centers serving patients with history of stroke, orthopedic joint replacement, heart failure, chronic

obstructive pulmonary disease, chronic kidney disease, acute myocardial infarction, diabetes, ventricular assist device implantation, stroke rehabilitation, cancer, asthma, and pneumonia, among others
- Centers/programs offering palliative care for adult and pediatric patients with serious illness

Manuals outlining guidelines are available for purchase at: http://store.jcrinc.com/publications/manuals

Guidelines and The Standard of Care: National Patient Safety Goals

What are the National Patient Safety Goals?

In 2002, The Joint Commission established its National Patient Safety Goals (NPSGs) program; the first set of NPSGs was effective January 1, 2003. The NPSGs were established to help accredited organizations address specific areas of concern in regards to patient safety.

How were the goals developed?

A panel of recognized patient safety experts called the Patient Safety Advisory Group advise the Joint Commission on the development and updating of NPSGs. The panel is composed of health care providers such as nurses, pharmacists, physicians, risk managers, and clinical engineers who are knowledgeable in addressing patient safety issues across multiple health care settings.

The Advisory Group recognizes evolving patient safety issues and advises the Joint Commission on how to address those issues through the NPSGs, and other venues such as their publication, *Sentinel Event Alerts*, standards and survey processes, performance measures, and educational materials. Following input from stakeholders (e.g. practitioners, provider organizations, purchasers, consumer groups), the Joint Commission defines the highest priority patient safety issues and best practices in addressing them. **Table 15** lists patient safety goals and examples.

Table 15. National Patient Safety Goals and Examples	
Goal Focus	*Examples*
Ambulatory Care	• Identify patients correctly • Use medicines safely • Prevent infection • Prevent mistakes in surgery
Behavioral Health Care	• Identify individuals correctly • Use medicine safely • Prevent infection • Identify individuals served safety risks
Critical Access Hospital	• Identify patients correctly • Improve staff communication • Use medicines safely • Use alarms safely • Prevent infection • Prevent mistakes in surgery
Home Care	• Identify patients correctly • Use medicines safely • Prevent infection • Prevent patients from falling • Identify patient safety risks
Hospital	• Identify patients correctly • Improve staff communication • Use medicines safely • Use alarms safely • Prevent infection • Identify patient safety risks • Prevent mistakes in surgery

§

References

Ambulatory Care National Patient Safety Goals http://www.jointcommission.org/assets/1/6/2014_AHC_NPSG_E.pdf

Behavioral Health National Patient Safety Goals http://www.jointcommission.org/assets/1/6/2014_BHC_

NPSG_E.pdf

Critical Access Hospital National Patient Safety Goals http://www.jointcommission.org/assets/1/6/2014_CAH_NPSG_E.pdf

Home Care National Patient Safety Goals http://www.jointcommission.org/assets/1/6/2014_OME_NPSG_E.pdf

Hospital National Patient Safety Goals http://www.jointcommission.org/assets/1/6/2014_HAP_NPSG_E.pdf

Tabers Online, 2000-2014, Unbound Medicine, Inc.

Resources

The Joint Commission Monographs and Papers
http://www.jointcommission.org/topics/monographs_
and_white_papers.aspx

The Joint Commission Sentinel Event
http://www.jointcommission.org/sentinel_event.aspx

7

CANCER-RELATED GUIDELINES AND THE STANDARD OF CARE: INTRODUCTION

WHAT HAVE WE COVERED SO FAR?

We have covered the foundational components of cancer care, symptom management, integrative oncology, and guideline development. We are now ready to introduce cancer-related guidelines.

WHO DETERMINES THE STANDARD OF CARE IN ONCOLOGY?

Oncology care guidelines are developed and disseminated by federal agencies, professional societies, associations, and academic groups. Some of these are listed below:

- American Cancer Society (ACS)
- American Society for Clinical Oncology (ASCO)

- American Society for Radiation Oncology (ASTRO)
- Children's Oncology Group (COG)
- European Society for Medical Oncology (ESMO)
- Multinational Association for Supportive Care in Cancer (MASCC)
- The National Cancer Institute (NCI)
- The National Comprehensive Cancer Network (NCCN
- Oncology Nursing Society (ONS)
- Society of Gynecologic Oncology (SGO)
- US Preventive Services Task Force (USPSTF)

Simply the development and publication of a guidelines or series of guidelines by any one group or organization *does not imply that* the standard is universally accepted nor does it imply that *all patients with that particular cancer would benefit from using the guideline.*

WHAT IS CANCER OVERDIAGNOSIS?

The goals of cancer awareness and screening are to reduce the rate of late-stage disease and decrease cancer mortality. Recent data has shown that these goals have not been met; rather, while there have been increases in detection of early-stage cancer, there is not a relative decline in detection of later-stage disease. Additionally, trends reveal that in some situations, cancer has been overdiagnosed, namely, situations where tumors are detected that would *not become* clinically apparent or cause death. Overdiagnosis may possibly lead to overtreatment.

Public data compiled by the Surveillance, Epidemiology, and End Results Program (SEER, National Cancer Institute) between 1975 and 2010 show three dominant patterns as a result of increased cancer screening and detection efforts:

- Screening has led to questionable significance in reducing overall rate of cancer occurrence.
- Yes, screening of cancer and removal of tumor has reduced incidence of this cancer and late-stage disease.
- No, screening of this pre-cancerous condition has not led to lower incidence of invasive cancer.

Table 16 lists tumor types, detection rates, and the clinical significance in changes brought about through screening.

Table 16. Cancer Screening Detection Rates and Clinical Significance by Tumor Type		
Tumor Type or Condition	*Detection Rates*	*Clinical Significance*
Breast Cancer	Increased	Screening has led to questionable significance in reducing overall rate of occurrence
Prostate Cancer	Increased	Screening has led to questionable significance in reducing overall rate of occurrence
Lung Cancer	Increased	Screening has led to detection of cancer with clinical significance if high-risk screening is adopted
Colon Cancer	Increased	Yes, screening of cancer and removal of tumor has reduced incidence of this cancer and late-stage disease
Cervical Cancer	Increased	Yes, screening of cancer and removal of tumor has reduced incidence of this cancer and late-stage disease
Barrett's esophagus (pre-cancerous condition)	Increased	No, screening of this pre-cancerous condition has not led to lower incidence of invasive cancer
Ductal carcinoma (DCIS, pre-cancerous condition)	Increased	No, screening of this pre-cancerous condition has not led to lower incidence of invasive cancer

❧

Reference

Howlader N, Noone AM, Krapcho M, Garshell J, Neyman N, Altekruse SF, Kosary CL, Yu M, Ruhl J, Tatalovich Z, Cho H, Mariotto A, Lewis DR, Chen HS, Feuer EJ, Cronin KA (eds). SEER Cancer Statistics Review, 1975-2010, National Cancer Institute. Bethesda, MD, http://seer.cancer.gov/csr/1975_2010/, based on November 2012 SEER data submission, posted to the SEER web site, April 2013.

To access this report: http://seer.cancer.gov/csr/1975_2010/sections.html. All material in this report is in the public domain and may be reproduced or copied without permission; citation as to source is above.

8

Cancer Screening Guidelines by Tumor Type: Introduction

How do screening tests become standard tests?

Evidence on the safety, accuracy, and usefulness of a cancer screening test is determined by different types of research studies. When enough evidence is available to demonstrate safety, accuracy, and usefulness of a test, the screening test then becomes a *standard* test. The different types of research studies used are randomized controlled trials, nonrandomized controlled trials, cohort studies, case-control studies, and ecologic studies (See Appendix A3 for explanations on each of these study types). Expert opinions (individuals or panels) by those knowledgeable in the field may also be included.

WHO ARE SOME OF THE LEADERS IN COMPILING, DEFINING, AND DISSEMINATING SCREENING GUIDELINES?

The American Cancer Society, National Cancer Institute, National Comprehensive Cancer Network, and the US Preventive Services Task Force are some the leading health organizations in compiling, defining and disseminating cancer screening guidelines in the US. These guidelines are designed for the screening of an asymptomatic population or in some cases, pre-identified high risk populations. Multiple health organizations and professional societies offer screening guidelines based on evidence-based summaries and clinical trials not represented here. Individuals seeking screening for common cancers should consult with their HCP on a regular basis regarding the appropriate validated screening tools recommended for their age group and medical status.

The Children's Oncology Group has developed follow-up guidelines for screening guidelines for survivors of childhood, adolescent, and young adult cancers, and these are included here as well.

Breast, cervical, colorectal, lung, and prostate cancers are the tumor types held in common for which screening guidelines and recommendations are compiled and disseminated across the leading health organizations.

As with other guidelines for cancer screening, we can expect that these guidelines will be revised as new research and clinical data become available. **Table 17** lists the leading health organizations and screening guidelines developed by tumor type.

Table 17. Leading Health Organizations Compiling and Disseminating Cancer Screening Guidelines and Recommendations by Tumor Type

	ACS	NCI	NCCN	USPSTF
Bladder		x		x
Breast	x	x	x	x
Cervical	x	x	x	x
Colorectal	x	x	x	x
Endometrial	x	x		
Esophageal		x		
Gastric		x		
Lung	x	x	x	x
Neuroblastoma		x		
Oral		x		x
Ovarian		x		x
Pancreatic		x		x
Prostate	x	x	x	x
Skin		x		x
Testicular		x		x

Acronyms:
ACS: American Cancer Society
NCI: National Cancer Institute
NCCN: National Comprehensive Cancer Network
USPSTF: US Preventive Services Task Force

COLLEEN O. LEE

§

References

American Cancer Society http://www.cancer.org/healthy/
findcancerearly/cancerscreeningguidelines/american-
cancer-society-guidelines-for-the-early-detection-of-
cancer

The National Cancer Institute Screening-Related
Guideline
http://www.cancer.gov/cancertopics/screening

The National Comprehensive Cancer Network Screening-
Related Guidelines http://www.nccn.org/professionals/
physician_gls/f_guidelines.asp#detection

US Preventive Services Task Force Screening-Related
Guidelines http://www.uspreventiveservicestaskforce.org/
uspstopics.htm

Children's Oncology Group Screening-Related Guidelines
Long-Term Follow-Up Guidelines for Survivors of
Childhood, Adolescent, and Young Adult Cancers: screen-
ing for survivors http://www.survivorshipguidelines.org/

9

Breast Cancer Screening Guidelines

Introduction

Breast cancer is the most frequently diagnosed cancer in U.S. women (excluding skin cancer). An estimated 232,670 new cases of invasive disease, 62, 570 cases of in situ disease, and 40,000 deaths are expected in 2014. In men, 2360 new cases and 430 deaths are expected. (American Cancer Society, 2014).

Screening for breast cancer for women at average risk includes clinical breast exam (CBE) and mammography. Mammography can often detect early stage breast cancer and is the most widely used screening modality. CBE and breast self-exam (BSE) have been evaluated and are of unclear benefit. Technologies such as ultrasound, magnetic resonance imaging (MRI), breast tomosynthesis (3D mammography), and molecular breast imaging are being evaluated, usually as additions to mammography.

HOW SENSITIVE AND SPECIFIC
IS MAMMOGRAPHY?

The sensitivity of mammography refers to the percentage of breast cancers that are detected when breast cancer is actually present. Overall mammography sensitivity is about 79%. Many factors influence sensitivity such as tumor size, breast tissue density, age, timing within the menstrual cycle, mammography image quality, and the radiologists' skill level in interpreting the findings. Sensitivity is lower than 79% in younger women and those with dense breast tissue.

Specificity of mammography is its ability to provide a normal result (no cancer) in the absence of cancer, in this case, breast cancer. Conversely, a false-positive result is when cancer is detected in the absence of cancer. When specificity is low, there is an increased possibility of false positive results which may lead to unnecessary examinations and procedures.

ARE THERE FAMILIAL/HEREDITARY BREAST
CANCERS AND RELATED SYNDROMES?

Up to 10% of breast cancers are due to specific mutations in single genes that are passed down in a family (hereditary). Specific patterns of hereditary breast/ovarian cancers are linked to mutations in the *BRCA 1* or *BRCA 2* genes. In addition, two very rare hereditary cancer syndromes showing an creased risk of breast cancer are Li-Fraumeni syndrome and Cowden syndrome. These syndromes are related to the 'germline' mutations in the *TP53* and *PTEN* genes respectively. A 'germline mutation' is a change in the gene in a body's egg or sperm that becomes part of the DNA of every cell in the body of the offspring and also known as 'hereditary mutation' (National Cancer Institute, 2014). The risk of developing cancer in individuals with one of these hereditary syndromes depends upon many variables (lifestyle factors, age, gender, among others).

Li-Fraumeni syndrome is associated with a high life-time risk of cancer such as soft-tissue sarcoma, osteosarcoma, premenopausal breast cancer, acute leukemia, and cancer of the colon, adrenal cortex, and brain tumors.

Cowden syndrome is another rate hereditary cancer syndrome associated with multiple cancerous lesions in the skin, mucous membranes, breast, thyroid, endometrium, and brain. Women diagnosed with Cowden syndrome have a high risk of benign fibrocystic breast disease, and their lifetime risk of breast cancer is 25-50% with an average age of 38-46 years at diagnosis (NCCN, 2014 Genetic/ Familial High-Risk Assessment: Breast and Ovarian).

Table 18 reviews breast cancer screening guidelines from four of the leading health organizations: ACS, NCI, NCCN, and USPSTF.

Acronyms in Table 18:

BSE: breast self-exam

CBE: clinical breast exam

HCP: health care provider

LFS: Li-Fraumeni syndrome

MRI: magnetic resonance imaging

Table 18. Breast Cancer Screening Guidelines

American Cancer Society

- Recommends yearly mammograms starting at age 40 and continuing for as long as a woman is in good health.
- Recommends CBE about every 3 years for women in their 20s and 30s and every year for women 40 and over.
- Recommends that women know how their breasts normally look and feel and report any breast changes promptly to their HCP. BSE is an option for women starting in their 20s.
- Recommends that some women should be screened with MRI in addition to mammograms (family history, a genetic tendency, or certain other factors may suggest this).
- Recommends against MRI screening for women whose lifetime risk of breast cancer is less than 15%.

Reference
http://www.cancer.org/cancer/breastcancer/moreinformation/breastcancerearlydetection/breast-cancer-early-detection-acs-recs

National Cancer Institute

- Recommends the use of screening mammography as it has solid evidence of benefit for women aged 40 to 70 years.
- Does not recommend CBE as a screening modality when it is used alone versus usual care
- Does not recommend the use of BSE alone as it has not been shown to reduce breast cancer mortality
- Recommends the use of MRI in women with a high risk of breast cancer

Reference
http://www.cancer.gov/cancertopics/pdq/screening/breast/healthprofessional

---

National Comprehensive Cancer Network

- Recommend annual MRI screening for individuals with BRCA mutation, 1st degree relative of BRCA carrier (but untested), and lifetime risk ~20% or greater (as defined by BRCAPRO or other models dependent on family history) (4).
- Recommend annual MRI screening for individuals with prior radiation to chest between age 10 to 20 years, Li-Fraumini syndrome and 1st degree relatives, Cowden and Bannayan-Riley-Ruvalcaba syndromes and 1st degree relatives (5,6).
- Current evidence is insufficient to recommend for or against MRI screening for individuals with lifetime risk 15-20% as defined by BRCAPRO or other models dependent on family history, LCIS or atypical lobular hyperplasia, atypical ductal hyperplasia, heterogeneously or extremely dense breast on mammography, or women with a personal history of breast cancer, including ductal carcinoma in situ (7).

- Recommend no MRI screening for women at < 15% lifetime risk (5).

References:
BRCAPRO: Breast cancer risk model (statistical model with associated software at http://bcb.dfci.harvard.edu/bayesmendel/brcapro.php

Saslow, D., Boetes, C., Burke, W., Harms, S., Leach, M. O., Lehman, C. D., . . . Russell, C. A. (2007). American Cancer Society guidelines for breast screening with MRI as an adjunct to mammography. CA Cancer J Clin, 57(2), 75-89.

Numerical references:
(4) Evidence from nonrandomized screening trails and observational studies
(5) Based on evidence of lifetime risk for breast cancer
(6) There is variation in recommendations for initiation of screening for different genetic syndromes.
(7) Screening decisions should be completed on a case-by-case basis.

http://www.nccn.org/professionals/physician_gls/f_guidelines.asp#detection

NCCN (2014) http://www.nccn.org/professionals/physician_gls/pdf/genetics_screening.pdf
[Genetic/Familial High-Risk Assessment: Breast and Ovarian; Version 1.2014, 2/28/2014]

US Preventive Services Task Force *
- Recommends biennial screening mammography for women aged 50 to 74 years (Grade B recommendation).
- Decision to begin biennial screening mammography before the age of 50 years is individual and should take patient context into account including values regarding benefits and harms (Grade: C recommendation).
- Current evidence is insufficient to assess the additional benefits and harms of screening mammography in women 75 years or older (Grade: I Statement).
- Recommends against teaching BSE (Grade: D recommendation).
- Current evidence is insufficient to assess the additional benefits and harms of CBE beyond screening mammography in women 40 years or older (Grade: I Statement).
- Current evidence is insufficient to assess the additional benefits and harms of either digital mammography or MRI instead of film mammography as screening modalities for breast cancer (Grade: I Statement).

Reference
http://www.uspreventiveservicestaskforce.org/uspstf/uspsbrca.htm The USPSTF is updating its recommendation on screening for breast cancer. It developed a research plan posted for public comment late 2013.

§

RELATED REFERENCES

American Cancer Society, *Cancer Facts & Figures 2014:* http://www.cancer.org/research/cancerfactsstatistics/cancerfactsfigures2014/index.

Elmore, J. G., & Kramer, B. S. (2014). Breast cancer screening: Toward informed decisions. JAMA, 311(13), 1298-1299. doi: 10.1001/jama.2014.2494

Mitka, M. (2013). Physicians, patients not following advice from USPSTF on mammography screening. JAMA, 309(20), 2084-2084. doi: 10.1001/jama.2013.5951

National Cancer Institute

Breast Cancer Screening Concepts http://www.cancer.gov/cancertopics/pdq/screening/breast/healthprofessional/page4

Breast Cancer Surveillance Consortium http://breastscreening.cancer.gov/

Germline Mutation http://www.cancer.gov/dictionary?CdrID=46384

Pace, L. E., & Keating, N. L. (2014). A systematic assessment of benefits and risks to guide breast cancer screening decisions. JAMA, 311(13), 1327-1335. doi: 10.1001/jama.2014.1398

Shimkin, M. B. (2014). Screening by mammography. JAMA, 311(13), 1362-1362. doi: 10.1001/jama.2013.279425 Slomski, A. (2014). Mammography no benefit in reducing deaths from breast cancer. JAMA, 311(12), 1191-1191. doi: 10.1001/jama.2014.3043

Susan G. Komen (2014). *Early Detection and Screening.* http://ww5.komen.org/breastcancer/earlydetectionampscreening.html

U.S. Preventive Services Task Force. Screening for Breast Cancer: Draft Research Plan. AHRQ Publication No.

14-05201-EF-5. http://www.uspreventiveservicestaskforce.org/uspstf14/breastcancer/breastcandraftresplan.htm

Walter, L. C., & Schonberg, M. A. (2014). Screening mammography in older women: A review. JAMA, 311(13), 1336-1347. doi: 10.1001/jama.2014.2834

10

CERVICAL CANCER SCREENING GUIDELINES

INTRODUCTION

Cervical cancer will account for an estimated 12,360 new cases of invasive disease and 4020 deaths in 2014. The incidence and mortality associated with cervical cancer has declined in recent decades due to prevention and early detection related to the Papanicolaou (Pap) test's ability to detect precancerous lesions (American Cancer Society, 2014). The benefits of screening women younger than 21 years are lesser because of low frequency of lesions that can grow to invasive cancer. Screening is not useful in women older than 65 years if they have had a history of recent negative Pap tests. The Pap test is the most widely used screening tests for cervical cancer with a greater than 80% magnitude of effect (National Cancer Institute, 2014).

In 2012, health organizations issued new cervical cancer screening guidelines that extend the time interval between screening tests for most women. Based on comprehensive reviews of available data, including NCI-funded research, the new guidelines seek to maximize the benefits of current screening tests while minimizing their potential harms. The USPSTF released one set of guidelines (Moyer, 2012), and a group of three health organizations, namely the American Cancer Society (ACS), the American Society for Colposcopy and Cervical Pathology (ASCCP), and the American Society for Clinical Pathology (ASCP) collaborated on the release of a second set (Saslow, et.al., 2012). Although the two sets of guidelines were developed independently, their recommendations are consistent.

Table 19 reviews cervical cancer screening guidelines from four of the leading health organizations: ACS, NCI, NCCN, and USPSTF.

Acronyms in Table 19:

HCP: Health care provider
HPV: human papilloma virus test
PAP: Pap test, Pap smear, Papanicolaou test

Table 19. Cervical Cancer Screening Guidelines

American Cancer Society

- Recommends screening begins at age 21. Women between ages 21 and 29 should have a Pap test every 3 years. HPV test may be used after an abnormal Pap test.
- Recommends Pap test plus an HPV test for women between ages of 30 and 65 every 5 years. This is the preferred approach, but it is also acceptable to have a Pap test alone every 3 years.
- Recommends no annual PAP test for women of any age by any screening method.
- Recommends women who are at high risk of cervical cancer because of a suppressed immune system (e.g. HIV infection, organ transplant, long term steroid use, or exposure to DES in utero) may need screening more often and should follow the recommendations of their HCP.
- Recommends no more PAP tests for women over age 65 who have had regular cervical cancer testing with normal results. Women with a history of a serious cervical pre-cancer should continue to be tested for at least 20 years after that diagnosis, even if testing continues past age 65.
- Recommends no more PAP tests for women who have had their cervix and uterus removed for reasons not related to cervical cancer and who have no history of cervical cancer or serious pre-cancer.
- Recommends women who have been vaccinated against HPV should still follow the screening recommendations for her age group.

Reference
http://www.cancer.org/cancer/cervicalcancer/moreinformation/cervicalcancerpreventionandearlydetection/cervical-cancer-prevention-and-early-detection-find-pre-cancer-changes

National Cancer Institute supports the joint guidelines developed by the American Cancer Society (ACS), American Society for Colposcopy and Cervical Pathology (ASCCP), American Society for Clinical Pathology (ASCP) along with the USPSTF recommendation statement.

References National Cancer Institute, "Leading Health Organizations Revision Cervical Cancer Screening Guidelines" http://www.cancer.gov/ncicancerbulletin/032012/page2

Saslow, D., Solomon, D., Lawson, H. W., Killackey, M., Kulasingam, S. L., Cain, J., . . . Myers, E. R. (2012). American Cancer Society, American Society for Colposcopy and Cervical Pathology, and American Society for Clinical Pathology screening guidelines for the prevention and early detection of cervical cancer. CA Cancer J Clin, 62(3), 147-172. doi: 10.3322/caac.21139

National Comprehensive Cancer Network supports the joint guidelines developed by the American Cancer Society (ACS), American Society for Colposcopy and

Cervical Pathology (ASCCP), American Society for Clinical Pathology (ASCP).

References Saslow, D., Solomon, D., Lawson, H. W., Killackey, M., Kulasingam, S. L., Cain, J., . . . Myers, E. R. (2012). American Cancer Society, American Society for Colposcopy and Cervical Pathology, and American Society for Clinical Pathology screening guidelines for the prevention and early detection of cervical cancer. Am J Clin Pathol, 137(4), 516-542. doi: 10.1309/ajcptgd94evrsjcg

Saslow, D., Solomon, D., Lawson, H. W., Killackey, M., Kulasingam, S. L., Cain, J. M., . . . Waldman, J. (2012). American Cancer Society, American Society for Colposcopy and Cervical Pathology, and American Society for Clinical Pathology screening guidelines for the prevention and early detection of cervical cancer. J Low Genit Tract Dis, 16(3), 175-204. doi: 10.1097/LGT.0b013e31824ca9d5

US Preventive Services Task Force

- Recommends screening in women ages 21 to 65 years with Pap every 3 years or, for women ages 30 to 65 years who want to lengthen the screening interval, screening with a combination of cytology and HPV testing every 5 years (Grade: A Recommendation).

- Recommends no screening in women younger than age 21 years (Grade: D Recommendation).

- Recommends no screening in women older than age 65 years who have had adequate prior screening and are not otherwise at high risk for cervical cancer (Grade: D Recommendation).

- Recommends no screening in women who have had a hysterectomy with removal of the cervix and who do not have a history of a serious pre-cancer (Grade: D Recommendation).

- Recommends no screening with HPV testing, alone or in combination with Pap, in women younger than age 30 years (Grade: D Recommendation).

Reference Moyer, V. A. (2012). Screening for Cervical Cancer: U.S. Preventive Services Task Force Recommendation Statement. Annals of Internal Medicine, 156(12), 880-891. doi: 10.7326/0003-4819-156-12-201206190-00424

§

Related References

American Cancer Society, Cancer Facts & Figures 2014: http://www.cancer.org/research/cancerfactsstatistics/cancerfactsfigures2014/index

American Congress of Obstetricians and Gynecologists (2012). *New Cervical Cancer Screening Recommendations from the U.S. Preventive Services Task Force and the American Cancer Society/American Society for Colposcopy and Cervical Pathology/American Society for Clinical Pathology* https://www.acog.org/About_ACOG/Announcements/New_Cervical_Cancer_Screening_Recommendations

Feldman, S. (2014). Can the New Cervical Cancer Screening and Management Guidelines Be Simplified? JAMA Intern Med. doi: 10.1001/jamainternmed.2014.576

National Cancer Institute (2014). *Overview- Cervical Cancer Screening* http://www.cancer.gov/cancertopics/pdq/screening/cervical/HealthProfessional

11

Colorectal Cancer Screening Guidelines

Introduction

Colorectal cancer is the third most common cancer in men and women in the US. An estimated 96,830 new cases of colon cancer and 40,000 cases of rectal cancer are anticipated in 2014. The incidence of colorectal cancer has diminished in the past two decades due to an increased in screening for and the removal of polyps (American Cancer Society, 2014).

Regular screening can often find colorectal cancer early, when it is most likely to be curable. In many cases, screening can also prevent colorectal cancer altogether. This is because polyps can be found and removed before they have the chance to turn into cancer.

In March 2008, the American Cancer Society, the U.S. Multi-Society Task Force on Colorectal Cancer, and the American College of Radiology mutually recommended screening for colorectal cancer beginning at 50 years of age by 1) high-sensitivity FOBT or fecal immunochemical testing annually, 2) flexible sigmoidoscopy every 5 years, 3) double-contrast barium enema every 5 years, 4) CT colonography (virtual colonoscopy) every 5 years, 5) colonoscopy every 10 years, or 6) fecal DNA at a currently unspecified interval. The American College of Obstetricians and Gynecologists suggests screening via colonoscopy as the preferred method. The American College of Physicians, American Academy of Family Physicians, American College of Preventive Medicine, and Centers for Disease Control and Prevention have issued comparable recommendations or recognized the USPSTF recommendation.

Colorectal cancer often occurs sporadically but familial cancer syndromes are common. Familial syndromes are inherited and genetics-based. Well-defined familial syndromes are Lynch syndrome (also known an HNPCC), familial adenomatous polyposis (FAP), and MUTYH-associated polyposis (MAP). Other syndromes include Cowden, Peutz-Jeghers, Muir-Torre, Turcot, Gardnes, Bannayan-Riley-Ruvalcaba, juvenile polyposis, and serrated polyposis syndromes. Whenever concern exits regarding a hereditary syndrome, the guidelines recommend referral to a genetics counselor.

The lifetime risk for individuals with CRC who carry one of the Lynch Syndrome-associated genetic mutations approaches 80%. Intensive screening is recommended although the intervals for screening are updated as new information becomes available. Many cancer centers routinely test for LS-related genetic mutations on all newly-diagnosed colorectal and endometrial cancers regardless of family history. Other cancer centers adopt an alternative approach and test all newly-diagnosed CRC patients less than 70 years of age and meet Bethesda criteria (Umar, et al, 2004). Genetic counseling combined with surveillance for high risk HNPCC family members should begin at age 25 (Kouraklis & Misiakos, 2005).

Table 20 reviews colorectal cancer screening guidelines from four of the leading health organizations: ACS, NCI, NCCN, and USPSTF.

Acronyms in Table 20:
CRC: colorectal cancer
CT: computed tomography scan
CTC: computer tomography colonography (virtual colonoscopy)
DCBE: double-contrast barium enema
FAP: familial adenomatous polyposis
FIT: fecal immunochemical test (also known as iFOBT with "I" = immunochemical or immunohistochemical)
FOBT: high-sensitivity fecal occult blood tests

HNPCC: hereditary nonpolyposis colorectal cancer
LS: Lynch Syndrome
MAP: *MUTYH*-Associated Polyposis

Table 20. Colorectal Cancer Screening Guidelines

American Cancer Society

- Recommends tests that detect both polyps and cancer: (1) Flexible sigmoidoscopy every 5 years* or colonoscopy every 10 years, (2) DCBE every 5 years* or (3) CTC every 5 years*.

- Recommends tests that primarily find cancer: Yearly FOBT or yearly FIT every year*,**

* If the test is positive, a colonoscopy should be done.
** The multiple stool take-home test should be used. One test performed in the office is not adequate for testing. A colonoscopy should be performed if the test is positive.

Reference: http://www.cancer.org/cancer/colonandrectumcancer/detailedguide/colorectal-cancer-detection. Site last revised 1/31/2014.

National Cancer Institute supports the USPSTF in strongly recommending screening for colorectal cancer in individuals at average risk at regular intervals with FOBT, sigmoidoscopy, or colonoscopy beginning at age 50. Individuals at increased risk because of a family history of colorectal cancer or polyps (or inflammatory bowel disease or certain inherited conditions) may be advised to start screening before age 50 and/or have more frequent screening.

Reference
http://www.cancer.gov/cancertopics/factsheet/detection/colorectal-screening. Site last updated 12/19/2013

National Comprehensive Cancer Network

Screening tests that detect adenomatous polyps and cancer

- Colonoscopy every 10 years for average-risk individuals; shorter intervals may be indicated based on quality and completeness of the colonoscopy; the number and characteristic of the polyps as well as family history and medical assessment should be taken into account

- Flexible sigmoidoscopy every 5 years; may be performed alone in combination with stool-based screening

- CTC every 5 years

Screening tests that primarily detect cancer

- Stool-based screening: (a) guaiac-based testing annually, (b) FIT/iFOBT, (c) stool DNA test with high sensitivity

For increased risk based on positive family history

- 1st degree relative with CRC aged < 50 years or two first degree relatives with CRC at any age:

    - Colonoscopy at age 40years or 10years before earliest diagnosis of CRC then repeat every 3-5 years depending on individual family history

- 1st degree relative with CRC aged ≥ 50 years:

    - Colonoscopy beginning at age 50 years or 10 years before earliest diagnosis of CRC then repeat every 5 years

- One 2nd degree relative with CRC aged < 50 years

    - Colonoscopy beginning at age 50 years then repeat per colonoscopy findings

- 1st degree relative with advanced adenoma(s)

    - Colonoscopy beginning at age 50 years or at age of onset, whichever is first then repeat per colonoscopy findings

For high-risk syndromes:

- Recommend either (a) testing all newly-diagnosed CRC individuals < 70 years plus individuals diagnosed at older ages meeting the Bethesda criteria or (b) universal testing of all newly-diagnosed CRC individuals less than 70 years of age for Lynch syndrome [HNPCC] other polyposis syndromes*

- Cowden Syndrome**

- Li-Fraumeni Syndrome**

Reference

http://www.nccn.org/professionals/physician_gls/f_guidelines.asp#detection. Site last updated 7/1/2013

* http://www.nccn.org/professionals/physician_gls/pdf/genetics_colon.pdf [Genetic/Familial High-Risk Assessment: Colorectal Cancer; Version 1.2014, 2/24/2014]

** http://www.nccn.org/professionals/physician_gls/pdf/genetics_screening.pdf [Genetic/Familial High-Risk Assessment: Breast and Ovarian; Version 1.2014, 2/28/2014]

US Preventive Services Task Force

- Recommends screening using fecal occult blood testing, sigmoidoscopy, or colonoscopy, in adults, beginning at age 50 years and continuing until age 75 years (Grade: A Recommendation).

- Recommends no screening in adults age 76 to 85 years (Grade: C

Recommendation).

- Recommends no screening in adults older than age 85 years (Grade: D Recommendation).

- Concludes that evidence is insufficient to assess the benefits and harms of computed tomographic colonography and fecal DNA testing as screening modalities for colorectal cancer (Grade: I Statement).

Reference

Whitlock, E. P., Lin, J. S., Liles, E., Beil, T. L., & Fu, R. (2008). Screening for Colorectal Cancer: A Targeted, Updated Systematic Review for the U.S. Preventive Services Task Force. Annals of Internal Medicine, 149(9), 638-658. doi: 10.7326/0003-4819-149-9-200811040-00245

§

RELATED REFERENCES

American Cancer Society, *Cancer Facts & Figures 2014:* http://www.cancer.org/research/cancerfactsstatistics/cancerfactsfigures2014/index

Inadomi, J. M. (2012). Why you should care about screening flexible sigmoidoscopy. N Engl J Med, 366(25), 2421-2422. doi: 10.1056/NEJMe1204099

Kastrinos, F., & Syngal, S. (2012). Screening patients with colorectal cancer for Lynch syndrome: what are we waiting for? J Clin Oncol, 30(10), 1024-1027. doi: 10.1200/jco.2011.40.7171

Kouraklis, G., & Misiakos, E. P. (2005). Hereditary non-polyposis colorectal cancer (Lynch syndrome): criteria for identification and management. Dig Dis Sci, 50(2), 336-344.

Qaseem, A., Denberg, T. D., Hopkins, R. H., Jr., Humphrey, L. L., Levine, J., Sweet, D. E., & Shekelle, P. (2012). Screening for colorectal cancer: a guidance statement from the American College of Physicians. Ann Intern Med, 156(5), 378-386. doi: 10.7326/0003-4819-156-5-201203060-00010

Siegel, R., Desantis, C., & Jemal, A. (2014). Colorectal cancer statistics, 2014. CA Cancer J Clin, 64(2), 104-117. doi: 10.3322/caac.21220

Sugerman, D. (2013). Options for colorectal cancer screening. JAMA, 310(6), 658-658. doi: 10.1001/jama.2013.57593

Too many US adults still pass up colorectal cancer screening. (2014). JAMA, 311(1), 20-20. doi: 10.1001/jama.2013.284165

Umar, A., Boland, C. R., Terdiman, J. P., Syngal, S., de la Chapelle, A., Ruschoff, J., . . . Srivastava, S. (2004). Revised Bethesda Guidelines for hereditary nonpolyposis colorectal cancer (Lynch syndrome) and microsatellite instability. J Natl Cancer Inst, 96(4), 261-268.

Zauber, A. G., Lansdorp-Vogelaar, I., Knudsen, A. B., Wilschut, J., van Ballegooijen, M., & Kuntz, K. M. (2008). Evaluating test strategies for colorectal cancer screening: a decision analysis for the U.S. Preventive Services Task Force. Ann Intern Med, 149(9), 659-669.

12

Lung Cancer Screening Guidelines

Introduction

Lung cancer is the most common cause of cancer death in men and women in the US. An estimated 224, 210 new cases of lung cancer are anticipated in 2014. The incidence of lung cancer has diminished since the mid 1980's in men but only since the mid-2000's in women. The incidence of lung cancer is low before the age of 50 years and increases afterward and especially after age 60 years. Lung cancer mortality rates are similar in magnitude to lung cancer incidence rates due to the high fatality rate from this disease. Most lung cancers are classified as non-small cell lung cancer (~85%); the remained is small cell lung cancer (~15%). Adenocarcinoma is the most common type of non-small cell lung cancer, and generally, screening guidelines mainly refer to the detection of adenocarcinoma (American Cancer Society, 2014).

The ACS joined with the American Society of Clinical Oncology, the American College of Chest Physicians, and the National Comprehensive Cancer Network to develop a systematic review (SR) following the announcement of the National Lung Screening Trial results in late 2010. The results from this trial showed 20% fever lung cancer deaths in current and former heavy smokers screened with spiral CT as compared to CXR. The joint SR evaluated the evidence on screening for lung cancer with low-dose CT scanning (LDCT). The focus was specifically on the potential benefits and harms of screening individuals who are at high risk of developing lung cancer, groups likely to benefit or not benefit from screening, and in what setting(s) is screening possibly effective (Wender, et.al 2013).

Overall, adults seeking testing for early lung cancer detection must be informed that screening will not detect all lung cancers, and the detection of a cancer by LDCT does not guarantee that death from lung cancer will be avoided.

Table 21 reviews lung cancer screening guidelines from four of the leading health organizations: ACS, NCI, NCCN, and USPSTF.

Acronyms in Table 21:

CT: computed tomography
LDCT: low dose CT scanning

Table 21. Lung Cancer Screening Guidelines

American Cancer Society

- Recommends no tests to screen for lung cancer in individuals who are at average risk of the disease.

- Recommends screening for individuals who are at high risk of lung cancer due to cigarette smoking meeting all of the following criteria: (1) 55 to 74 years of age, (2) in fairly good health, (3) at least a 30 pack-year smoking history AND are either is still smoking or has quit smoking within the last 15 years.

Reference:
Wender, R., Fontham, E. T., Barrera, E., Jr., Colditz, G. A., Church, T. R., Ettinger, D. S., Smith, R. A. (2013). American Cancer Society lung cancer screening guidelines. CA Cancer J Clin, 63(2), 107-117. doi: 10.3322/caac.21172.

National Cancer Institute

- Recommends screening by low-dose helical CT in people 55-74 years who have a history of smoking ≥ 30 pack years (1 pack per day for ≥30 years) and have quit within the last 15 years.

- Recommends no tests to screen for lung cancer in people who are at average risk of the disease

References:
Oken, M. M., Hocking, W. G., Kvale, P. A., Andriole, G. L., Buys, S. S., Church, T. R., Berg, C. D. (2011). Screening by chest radiograph and lung cancer mortality: the Prostate, Lung, Colorectal, and Ovarian (PLCO) randomized trial. JAMA, 306(17), 1865-1873. doi: 10.1001/jama.2011.1591

National Cancer Institute (2014). *Lung Cancer Screening: Evidence of Benefit Associated With Screening*.
http://www.cancer.gov/cancertopics/pdq/screening/lung/HealthProfessional

National Comprehensive Cancer Network

- Recommend that institutions performing lung cancer screening include the following specialties: thoracic radiology, pulmonary medicine, and thoracic surgery.

- Recommend baseline low-dose CT (LDCT) for high-risk individuals (category 1)

    o Age 55-74 and ≥ 30 pack year history of smoking who have stopped smoking < 15 years OR

- o Age ≥ 50 and ≥ 20 year pack year history of smoking and 1 additional risk factor (other than second hand smoke) (category 2B)

- o If no lung nodule is present, recommends annual LCDT for 2 years and consider annual LCDR until person no longer eligible for definitive treatment

- Recommend no tests to screen for lung cancer in individuals at moderate or low risk

  For moderate risk

  - o Age ≥ 50 years and ≥ 20 pack year history of smoking or second hand smoke exposure and no additional risk factors

  For low risk

  - o Age < 50 years and/or < 20 pack year smoking history

Reference:
NCCN Clinical Practice Guidelines in Oncology: Lung Cancer Screening, Version 2.2014: http://www.nccn.org/professionals/physician_gls/pdf/lung_screening.pdf

US Preventive Services Task Force

•The USPSTF recommends annual screening for lung cancer with low-dose computed tomography in adults ages 55 to 80 years who have a 30 pack-year smoking history and currently smoke or have quit within the past 15 years. Screening should be discontinued once a person has not smoked for 15 years or develops a health problem that substantially limits life expectancy or the ability or willingness to have curative lung surgery.

Grade: B recommendation.

Reference:
Screening for Lung Cancer: Recommendations from the U.S. Preventive Services Task Force. (2014). Annals of Internal Medicine, 160(5), I-40. doi: 10.7326/P14-9009

§

Related References

American Cancer Society, *Cancer Facts & Figures 2014:* http://www.cancer.org/research/cancerfactsstatistics/ cancerfactsfigures2014/index

de Koning, H. J., Meza, R., Plevritis, S. K., ten Haaf, K., Munshi, V. N., Jeon, J., . . . McMahon, P. M. (2014). Benefits and Harms of Computed Tomography Lung Cancer Screening Strategies: A Comparative Modeling Study for the U.S. Preventive Services Task Force. Annals of Internal Medicine, 160(5), 311-320. doi: 10.7326/ M13-2316

Harris, R. P., Sheridan, S. L., Lewis, C. L., & et al. (2014). The harms of screening: A proposed taxonomy and application to lung cancer screening. JAMA Intern Med, 174(2), 281-286. doi: 10.1001/jamainternmed.2013.12745

Humphrey, L. L., Deffebach, M., Pappas, M., Baumann, C., Artis, K., Mitchell, J. P., . . . Slatore, C. G. (2013). Screening for Lung Cancer With Low-Dose Computed Tomography: A Systematic Review to Update the U.S. Preventive Services Task Force Recommendation. Annals of Internal Medicine, 159(6), 411-420. doi: 10.7326/0003-4819-159-6-201309170-00690

Patz, E. F., Jr, Pinsky, P., Gatsonis, C., & et al. (2014). OVerdiagnosis in low-dose computed tomography screening for lung cancer. JAMA Intern Med, 174(2), 269-274. doi: 10.1001/jamainternmed.2013.12738

Tammemagi, M. C., Katki, H. A., Hocking, W. G., Church, T. R., Caporaso, N., Kvale, P. A., . . . Berg, C. D. (2013). Selection criteria for lung-cancer screening. N Engl J Med, 368(8), 728-736. doi: 10.1056/NEJMoa1211776

SUMMARIES FOR PATIENTS

American Cancer Society: Weight the Benefits and Risks of Lung Cancer Screening, Otis W. Brawley, MD: http://www.cancer.org/cancer/news/expertvoices/post/2013/01/11/weighing-the-benefits-and-risks-of-lung-cancer-screening.aspx

American Lung Association: Providing Guidance on Lung Cancer Screening to Patients and Physicians, April 23, 2012: http://www.lung.org/lung-disease/lung-cancer/lung-cancer-screening-guidelines/lung-cancer-screening.pdf

American Lung Association: Lung Cancer CT Screening: Is It Right for Me? http://www.lung.org/lung-disease/lung-cancer/lung-cancer-screening-guidelines/lung-cancer-screening-for-patients.pdf

Screening for Lung Cancer: Recommendations from the U.S. Preventive Services Task Force. (2014). Annals of Internal Medicine, 160(5), I-40. doi: 10.7326/P14-9009
NCCN Guidelines for Patients: Lung Cancer Screening Version 1.2014: http://www.nccn.org/patients/guidelines/lung_screening/index.html

13

Prostate Cancer Screening Guidelines

Introduction

Prostate cancer is the most frequently diagnosed cancer in men (aside from skin cancer). An estimated 223,000 new cases of prostate cancer are anticipated in 2014. The incidence of prostate cancer in African American men is about 60% higher than in non-Hispanic white men. The overall incidence rate from 2006 – 2010 has decreased by 2% yearly. Prostate cancer is now the second leading cause of cancer death in men surpassed only by lung cancer. Prostate cancer rarely causes death in men younger than 50 years. Most deaths associated with prostate cancer occur in men older than 75 years. Because of the potential for adverse effects associated with the treatment for prostate cancer and due to the tumors' slow-growing, non-lethal potential, presently, no national health organizations support regular prostate cancer screening (American Cancer Society, 2014).

The two most common screening tests for prostate cancer are the digital rectal examination (DRE) and the prostate-specific antigen (PSA). These screening tests are able to detect prostate cancer at an early stage, but it is not known whether this early detection (and possibly earlier treatment) leads to any adjustment in the natural history and outcome of the disease. In some situation, screening with PSA and/or DRE identifies some prostate cancers that would never have caused significant clinical complications.

Table 22 reviews prostate cancer screening guidelines from four of the leading health organizations: ACS, NCI, NCCN, and USPSTF. **Table 23** outlines the USPSTF Definition of the Grades and Practice Suggestions followed by **Table 24** describing the NCCN Categories of Evidence and Consensus

Acronyms in Table 22:
    DRE: digital rectal exam
    HCP: health care provider
    PSA: prostatic specific antigen

Table 22. Prostate Cancer Screening Guidelines

American Cancer Society

- Recommends that men make an informed decision with their doctor about whether to be tested for prostate cancer. Research has not yet proven that the potential benefits of testing outweigh the harms of testing and treatment.

- Recommends PSA blood test with or without a DRE starting at age 50 in men who are at average risk of prostate cancer and are expected to live at least 10 more years after talking with their HCP.

- Recommends discussion with HCP at age 40 for men at higher risk (those with more than one first-degree relative who had prostate cancer at an early age).

- Recommends that African American men who have a first-degree relative (father, brother, or son) diagnosed with prostate cancer at an early age (younger than age 65) should talk with their HCP starting at age 45.

- Assuming no prostate cancer is found as a result of screening, the time between future screenings depends on the results of the PSA blood test: (1) Men who choose to be tested who have a PSA of less than 2.5 ng/ml, may only need to be retested every 2 years and (2) Screening should be done yearly for men whose PSA level is 2.5 ng/ml or higher.

Reference:
http://www.cancer.org/cancer/prostatecancer/moreinformation/prostatecancerearlydetection/prostate-cancer-early-detection-acs-recommendations

National Cancer Institute

- Recommends against routine PSA-based and DRE-based screening for prostate cancer in men with average risk.

Reference: http://www.cancer.gov/cancertopics/pdq/screening/prostate/HealthProfessional

National Comprehensive Cancer Network

- Recommends against routine PSA-based and DRE-based screening for prostate cancer in men with average risk.

- Recommends repeat testing at 1-2 year intervals in men ages 45-49 years who have a normal DRE and PSA > 1ng/ml. Recommends repeat testing at age 50 for men ages 45-49 who have a normal DRE and PSA ≤ 1ng/ml (Category 2B).

- Recommends repeat testing at 1-2 year intervals in men age 50-70 years and men > 70 years with normal DRE, PSA < 3ng/ml and no other indications for biopsy (Category 2B).

Reference
NCCN Clinical Practice Guidelines in Oncology: Prostate Cancer Early Detection Version 1.
2014 http://www.nccn.org/professionals/physician_gls/pdf/prostate_detection.pdf

US Preventive Services Task Force

- Recommends against PSA-based screening for prostate cancer (Grade: D Recommendation).

  This recommendation applies to men in the general U.S. population, regardless of age but does not include PSA testing after diagnosis or treatment of prostate cancer.

- In October 2011, the USPSTF posted the draft of its recommendation regarding prostate cancer screening for public comment. "A better test and better treatment options are needed. Until these are available, the USPSTF has recommended against screening for prostate cancer."

Reference:
Screening for Prostate Cancer, Topic Page. U.S. Preventive Services Task Force.
http://www.uspreventiveservicestaskforce.org/prostatecancerscreening.htm. Site last revised:
07/01/2012

§

RELATED RESOURCES

American Cancer Society, Cancer Facts & Figures 2014: http://www.cancer.org/research/cancerfactsstatistics/cancerfactsfigures2014/index

American Urological Association, Detection of Prostate Cancer, *Early Detection of Prostate Cancer: AUA Guideline.* 2013 http://www.auanet.org/common/pdf/education/clinical-guidance/Prostate-Cancer-Detection.pdf
Basch, E., Oliver, T. K., Vickers, A., Thompson, I., Kantoff, P., Parnes, H., . . . Nam, R. K. (2012). Screening

for prostate cancer with prostate-specific antigen testing: American Society of Clinical Oncology Provisional Clinical Opinion. J Clin Oncol, 30(24), 3020-3025. doi: 10.1200/jco.2012.43.3441

Hayes, J. H., & Barry, M. J. (2014). Screening for prostate cancer with the prostate-specific antigen test: A review of current evidence. JAMA, 311(11), 1143-1149. doi: 10.1001/jama.2014.2085

Gulati, R., Gore, J. L., & Etzioni, R. (2013). Comparative Effectiveness of Alternative Prostate-Specific Antigen–Based Prostate Cancer Screening Strategies. Model Estimates of Potential Benefits and Harms. Annals of Internal Medicine, 158(3), 145-153. doi: 10.7326/0003-4819-158-3-201302050-00003

Moyer, V. A. (2012). Screening for Prostate Cancer: U.S. Preventive Services Task Force Recommendation Statement. Annals of Internal Medicine, 157(2), 120-134. doi: 10.7326/0003-4819-157-2-201207170-00459

Qaseem, A., Barry, M. J., Denberg, T. D., Owens, D. K., & Shekelle, P. (2013). Screening for Prostate Cancer: A Guidance Statement From the Clinical Guidlines Committee of the American College of Physicians. Annals of Internal Medicine, 158(10), 761-769. doi: 10.7326/0003-4819-158-10-201305210-00633

SUMMARY FOR PATIENTS

Screening Smarter, Not Harder, for Prostate Cancer. (2013). Annals of Internal Medicine, 158(3), I-30. doi: 10.7326/0003-4819-158-3-201302050-00001

NCCN Guidelines for Patients: Prostate Cancer http://www.nccn.org/patients/guidelines/prostate/index.html

Table 23. USPSTF Definition of the Grades and Practice Suggestions		
Grade	*Definition*	*Practice Suggestions*
A	Recommends the service. There is high certainty that the net benefit is substantial.	Offer or provide this service.
B	Recommends the service. There is high certainty that the net benefit is moderate or there is moderate certainty that the net benefit is moderate to substantial.	Offer or provide this service.
C	Recommends selectively offering or providing this service to individual patients based on professional judgment and patient preferences. There is at least moderate certainty that the net benefit is small.	Offer or provide this service only if other considerations support the offering or providing the service in an individual patient.
D	Recommends against the service. There is moderate or high certainty that the service has no net benefit or that the harms outweigh the benefits.	Discourage the use of this service.
I Statement	Current evidence is insufficient to assess the balance of benefits and harms of the service. Evidence is lacking, of poor quality, or conflicting, and the balance of benefits and harms cannot be determined.	If the service is offered, patients should understand the uncertainty about the balance of benefits and harms.
http://www.uspreventiveservicestaskforce.org/uspstf/grades.htm		

Table 24. NCCN Categories of Evidence and Consensus	
Category	**Consensus Statement**
1	There is no uniform NCCN consensus that the intervention is appropriate based on high-level evidence
2A	There is uniform NCCN consensus that the intervention is appropriate based on lower-level evidence
2B	There is NCCN consensus that the intervention is appropriate based on lower-level evidence
3	There is major NCCN disagreement that the intervention is appropriate based on any level of evidence
http://www.nccn.org/professionals/physician_gls/pdf/lung_screening.pdf	

References

Levin B, Lieberman DA, McFarland, et al. Screening and Surveillance for the Early Detection of Colorectal Cancer and Adenomatous Polyps, 2008: A Joint Guideline from the American Cancer Society, the US Multi-Society Task Force on Colorectal Cancer, and the American College of Radiology. CA Cancer J Clin. 2008;58.

Saslow D, Boetes C, Burke W, et al for the American Cancer Society Breast Cancer Advisory Group. American Cancer Society guidelines for breast screening with MRI as an adjunct to mammography. CA Cancer J Clin. 2007;57:75-89.

Saslow D, Solomon D, Lawson H, et al. American Cancer Society, American Society for Colposcopy and Cervical Pathology, and American Society for Clinical Pathology Screening Guidelines for the Prevention and Early Detection of Cervical Cancer. CA Cancer J Clin. 2012 May-Jun;62(3):147-72. Epub 2012 Mar 14.

Smith RA, Brooks D, Cokkinides V, Salsow D, Brawley OW. Cancer screening in the United States, 2013: A review of current American Cancer Society guidelines, current issues in cancer screening, and new guidance on cervical cancer screening and lung cancer screening. CA Cancer J Clin 2013, Mar-Apr;63:87-105. Accessed at http://onlinelibrary.wiley.com/doi/10.3322/caac.21174/full on April 23, 2013.

Wender R, Fontham E, Barrera E, et al. American Cancer Society lung cancer screening guidelines: CA Cancer Journal for Clinicians. 2013 Jan 11 [Epub ahead of print].

14

Cancer Treatment Guidelines by Tumor Type

What have we covered so far?

Thus far, we have covered the foundational components of cancer care, symptom management, integrative oncology, guideline development, and cancer-related guidelines for the major cancers with known screening interventions. One of the most, if not the most, expansive topic in cancer care is treatment. Treatment guidelines for disease and symptom management are offered by major health organizations with updates as new research is published and new technologies are developed.

COLLEEN O. LEE

Which groups have developed oncology treatment guidelines?

Multiple oncology health organizations across the US have developed authoritative guidelines on the treatment of one or more cancer types. Cancer treatment guidelines change over time based on new drug development, research findings, and patient/care-giver input on therapy tolerance. Entire volumes of medical texts and oncology websites chronicle treatment regimens. This chapter is dedicated to listing some of those organizations and the cancer types reflected in their published guidelines at the time of this printing. The organizations are:

- American Society for Clinical Oncology
- American Society for Radiation Oncology
- European Society for Medical Oncology
- National Cancer Institute
- National Comprehensive Cancer Network
- Society of Gynecologic Oncology Clinical Practice Statements

The <u>American Society for Clinical Oncology</u> has published guidelines for the following cancers:

- Breast cancer
- Gastrointestinal cancer
- Genitourinary cancer

- Head and Neck cancer
- Hematologic malignancies
- Lung cancer
- Melanoma

http://www.asco.org/quality-guidelines/guidelines

The <u>American Society for Radiation Oncology</u> has published guidelines for the following cancers:

- Breast cancer
- Brain tumors
- Genitourinary cancers
- Thoracic malignancies

https://www.astro.org/Clinical Practice/Guidelines/Index.aspx

The <u>European Society for Medical Oncology</u> has published guidelines for the following cancers:

- Breast cancer
- Cancers of unknown primary site
- CNS malignancies
- Endocrine cancers
- Gastrointestinal cancer
- Genitourinary cancers
- Gynecological cancers

- Head and neck cancer
- Hematologic malignancies
- Lung cancer
- Melanoma
- Neuroendocrine Tumors
- Sarcoma and GIST

http://www.esmo.org/Guidelines-Practice/
Clinical-Practice-Guidelines

The National Cancer Institute has published PDQ® cancer information summaries for the following adult cancers:

Acute Lymphoblastic Leukemia

Acute Myeloid Leukemia

Adrenocortical Carcinoma

AIDS-Related Lymphoma

Anal Cancer

Bile Duct Cancer

Bladder Cancer

Brain Tumors

Breast Cancer

Breast Cancer and Pregnancy

Breast Cancer (Male)

Carcinoma of Unknown Primary

Cervical Cancer

Chronic Lymphocytic Leukemia

Chronic Myelogenous Leukemia

ChronicMyeloproliferative Disorders

CNS Lymphoma

Colon Cancer

Endometrial Cancer

Esophageal Cancer

Extragonadal Germ Cell Tumors

Gallbladder Cancer

Gastric Cancer

Gastrointestinal Carcinoid Tumors

Gastrointestinal Stromal Tumors

Gestational Trophoblastic Disease

Hairy Cell Leukemia

Hodgkin Lymphoma

Hypopharyngeal Cancer

Intraocular Melanoma

Islet Cell Tumors

Kaposi Sarcoma

Langerhans Cell Histiocytosis

Laryngeal Cancer

Lip and Oral Cavity Cancer

Liver Cancer

Malignant Mesothelioma

Melanoma

Melanoma, Intraocular (Eye)

Merkel Cell Carcinoma

Multiple Myeloma and Other Plasma Cell Neoplasms

Mycosis Fungoides
Myelodysplastic
Syndromes
Nasopharyngeal Cancer
Neck Cancer with Occult
Primary
Non-Hodgkin Lymphoma,
Adult
Non-Small Cell Lung
Cancer
Oropharyngeal Cancer
Ovarian Epithelial Cancer
Ovarian Germ Cell Tumors
Ovarian Low Malignant
Potential Tumors
Pancreatic Cancer
Pancreatic
Neuroendocrine Tumors
Paraganglioma
Parathyroid Cancer
Penile Cancer
Pheochromocytoma
Pituitary Tumors
Prostate Cancer
Rectal Cancer
Renal Cell Cancer
Salivary Gland Cancer
Soft Tissue Sarcoma

Sézary Syndrome
Skin Cancer
(Nonmelanoma)
Small Cell Lung Cancer
Small Intestine Cancer
Testicular Cancer
Thymoma
Thyroid Cancer
Transitional Cell Cancer
Urethral Cancer
Uterine Sarcoma
Vaginal Cancer
Vulvar Cancer

PDQ®, or Physician Data Query is the NCI's information database on the latest published information on
cancer-related topics. PDQ® information summaries are
reviewed regularly and updated as new information becomes available.

http://www.cancer.gov/cancertopics/pdq/adulttreatment

The National Cancer Institute has published PDQ® cancer information summaries for the following pediatric
cancers:

Acute Lymphoblastic Leukemia
Acute Myeloid Leukemia
Adrenocortical Carcinoma
Astrocytomas
Atypical Teratoid
Basal Cell Carcinoma
Bladder Cancer
Brain Stem Glioma
Embryonal Tumors
Craniopharyngioma
Ependymoma
Breast Cancer
Bronchial Tumors
Carcinoid Tumors
Carcinoma of Unknown Primary
Cardiac Tumors
Cervical Cancer
Chordoma
Colorectal Cancer
Craniopharyngioma
Ependymoma
Esophageal Tumors
Esthesioneuroblastoma
Ewing Sarcoma
Extracranial Germ Cell Tumors

Gastric (Stomach) Cancer
Gastrointestinal Stromal Tumors
Germ Cell Tumors
Glioma
Head and Neck Cancer
Histiocytoma of Bone
Hodgkin Lymphoma
Kidney Tumors
Langerhans Cell Histiocytosis
Laryngeal Cancer
Liver Cancer
Lung Cancer
Non-Hodgkin Lymphoma
Malignant Fibrous
Melanoma
Mesothelioma
Midline Tract Carcinoma
Multiple Endocrine Neoplasia
Nasopharyngeal Cancer
Neuroblastoma
Oral Cancer,
Osteosarcoma
Ovarian Cancer
Pancreatic Cancer
Papillomatosis

Paraganglioma
Pheochromocytoma
Pleuropulmonary
Blastoma
Retinoblastoma
Rhabdomyosarcoma
Salivary Gland Cancer
Soft Tissue Sarcoma
Skin Cancer
Squamous Cell Carcinoma
Testicular Cancer
Thymoma
Thyroid Tumors
Vaginal Cancer
Wilms Tumor

http://www.cancer.gov/cancertopics/pdq/
pediatrictreatment

The <u>National Comprehensive Cancer Network</u> has published guidelines for the following cancers:

Acute Lymphoblastic
Leukemia
Acute Myeloid Leukemia
Anal Carcinoma
Bladder Cancer
Bone Cancer
Breast Cancer
Cancer of Unknown
Primary
Central Nervous System
Cancers
Cervical Cancer
Chronic Myelogenous
Leukemia
Colon/Rectal Cancer
Colon Cancer
Rectal Cancer
Cutaneous Melanoma
Endometrial Cancer
Esophageal and
Esophagogastric Junction
Cancers
Fallopian Tube Cancer
Gastric Cancer
Head and Neck Cancers
Hepatobiliary Cancers
Hodgkin Lymphoma
Kidney Cancer

Malignant Pleural
Mesothelioma
Melanoma
Multiple Myeloma/Other
Plasma Cell Neoplasms
Multiple Myeloma
Systemic Light Chain
Amyloidosis
Waldenström's
Macroglobulinemia /
Lymphoplasmacytic
Lymphoma
Myelodysplastic
Syndromes
Neuroendocrine Tumors
Non-Hodgkin's
Lymphomas
Non-Melanoma Skin
Cancers
Basal and Squamous Cell
Skin Cancers
Dermatofibrosarcoma
Protuberans
Merkel Cell Carcinoma
Non-Small Cell Lung
Cancer
Occult Primary
Ovarian Cancer

Pancreatic
Adenocarcinoma
Penile Cancer
Primary Peritoneal
Cancer
Prostate Cancer
Small Cell Lung Cancer
Soft Tissue Sarcoma
Testicular Cancer
Thymomas and Thymic
Carcinomas
Thyroid Carcinoma
Uterine Neoplasms

http://www.nccn.org/professionals/physician_gls/
f_guidelines.asp#site

The <u>Society of Gynecologic Oncology</u> has published clinical practice guidelines for the following cancers:

- Genetics
- Ovarian Cancer
- Cervical Cancer
- Endometrial Cancer

https://www.sgo.org/clinical-practice/guidelines/

15

CANCER SUPPORTIVE CARE GUIDELINES

INTRODUCTION

Multiple oncology health organizations across the US have developed authoritative supportive care guidelines. Supportive care guidelines, as with treatment guidelines, change over time based on new drug development for cancer-related symptoms, research findings, and patient/care-giver input on tolerance of individual interventions. Entire volumes of medical and nursing texts and oncology care websites chronicle supportive care best-practice interventions. This chapter is dedicated to listing some of those organizations and the symptoms reflected in their published guidelines at the time of this printing. The organizations are:

- American Society for Clinical Oncology
- Children's Oncology Group

- European Society for Medical Oncology
- Multinational Association for Supportive Care
- National Cancer Institute
- National Comprehensive Care Network
- Oncology Nursing Society

The <u>American Society for Clinical Oncology</u> has published guidelines on the following topics:

- Assays and predictive markers
- Supportive care and quality of life
- Survivorship
- Treatment-related issues

Quality Initiatives (Examples)

- ASCO-ONS Standards for Safe Chemotherapy Administration
- ASCO-NCCN Quality Measures
- Consensus Statement on Quality Cancer Care

http://www.asco.org/quality-guidelines/guidelines

The <u>Children's Oncology Group</u> has published guidelines on the following topics:

- Community Support
- School Support
- Grieving and Palliative Care
- Informed Consent

http://www.childrensoncologygroup.org/index.php/
coping-with-cancer-293

The <u>European Society for Medical Oncology Supportive Care</u> has published guidelines on the following topics:

- Cancer, pregnancy, and fertility
- Management of chemotherapy extravasation
- Cardiovascular toxicity induced by chemotherapy, targeted agents and radiotherapy
- Management of cancer pain
- Management of venous thromboembolism in cancer patients
- Management of oral and gastrointestinal mucositis
- Erythropoiesis-stimulating agents in the treatment of anemia in cancer patients
- Prevention of chemotherapy and radiotherapy-induced nausea and vomiting
- Management of febrile neutropenia
- Hematopoietic growth factors

http://www.esmo.org/Guidelines-Practice/
Clinical-Practice-Guidelines/Supportive-Care

The Multinational Association for Supportive Care
in Cancer has published guidelines on the following
topics:

- Mucositis Guidelines
- Antiemetic Guidelines
- Guideline for the Prevention of Acute Nausea
  and Vomiting due to Antineoplastic Medication
  in Pediatric Cancer Patients (partnership with
  Pediatric Oncology Group of Ontario)
- International Pediatric Fever and Neutropenia
  Guideline (partnership with The Hospital for Sick
  Children)
- MASCC Oral Agent Teaching Tool© (MOATT©)
- MASCC EGFR Inhibitor Skin Toxicity Tool
  (MESTT©)

http://www.mascc.org/practice-resources

The National Cancer Institute has published guidelines
on the following topics:

- Adjustment to Cancer: Anxiety and Distress
- Cardiopulmonary Syndromes

- Communication in Cancer Care
- Delirium
- Depression
- Family Caregivers in Cancer: Roles and Challenges
- Fatigue
- Gastrointestinal Complications
- Grief, Bereavement, and Coping with Loss
- Last Days of Life
- Lymphedema
- Late Effects Treatment for Childhood Cancer
- Nausea and Vomiting
- Nutritional in Cancer Care
- Oral Complications of Chemotherapy and Head/ Neck Radiation
- Pain
- Pediatric Supportive Care
- Post-traumatic Stress Disorder
- Pruritis
- Sexuality and Reproductive Issues
- Sleep Disorders
- Smoking in Cancer Care
- Spirituality in Cancer Care
- Sweats and Hot Flashes
- Transitional Care Planning

http://www.cancer.gov/cancertopics/pdq/supportivecare

The <u>National Comprehensive Care Network</u> has published guidelines on the following topics:

- Adolescent and Young Adult Oncology
- Adult Cancer Pain
- Antiemesis
- Cancer- and Chemotherapy-Induced Anemia
- Cancer-Related Fatigue
- Distress Management
- Myeloid Growth Factors
- Palliative Care
- Prevention and Treatment of Cancer-Related Infections
- Senior Adult Oncology
- Survivorship
- Venous Thromboembolic Disease

The <u>Oncology Nursing Society</u> has published guidelines on the following topics:

- Anorexia
- Anxiety
- Caregiver Strain and Burden
- Chemotherapy-Induced Nausea and Vomiting
- Cognitive Impairment
- Constipation
- Depression

- Diarrhea (Chemotherapy-Induced, Radiation–Induced)
- Dyspnea
- Fatigue
- Hot Flashes
- Lymphedema
- Mucositis
- Pain (Acute, Breakthrough, Chronic, Refractory/Intractable)
- Peripheral Neuropathy
- Prevention of Bleeding
- Prevention of Infection (General, Transplant)
- Radiodermatitis
- Skin Reactions
- Sleep-Wake Disturbances

https://www.ons.org/practice-resources/pep

Other ONS oncology-related topics are:

- Red Flags in Caring for Cancer Survivors

https://www.ons.org/sites/default/files/media/Red%20Flags%20for%20Cancer%20Survivors.pdf

- Standards of Oncology Education: Patient/Significant Other and Public https://www.ons.org/products/standards-oncology-education-patientsignificant-other-and-public-3rd-edition

- Standards of Oncology Nursing Education: Generalist and Advanced Practice Levels

https://www.ons.org/products/standards-oncology-nursing-education-generalist-and-advanced-practice-levels-third-edition

- Statement on the Scope and Standards of Oncology Nursing Practice: Generalist and Advanced Practice

https://www.ons.org/products/statement-scope-and-standards-oncology-nursing-practice-generalist-and-advanced-practice

16

Integrative Oncology Guidelines

Introduction
As reviewed in Chapter 4, complementary and/or alternative medicine (CAM) is traditional medicine combined with CAM approaches (complementary) or instead of (alternative) traditional approaches. Integrative oncology is the combination of integrative medicine and evidence-based oncology care. Integrative oncology focuses on a comprehensive health approach to the human body, mind, soul, and spirit throughout the cancer care spectrum.

The Society for Integrative Oncology
The Society for Integrative Oncology (SIO) is the professional association solely dedicated to the integration of CAM practice, education, and research into cancer care

SIO published its first iteration of evidence-based, clinical *Practice Guidelines for Integrative Oncology* in 2007 which were later amended and made public in 2009 (Deng et al., 2009). The guidelines are for clinicians to use when making clinical choices for their patients. Additionally, the guidelines may be useful for quality assurance, clinical decision-making, and may provide indications for reimbursement in clinical programs.

SIO emphasizes that the integrative oncology guidelines "*are tools, not rules,*" and clinical decision-making should be based on the best-available evidence, knowledge of the safety profile and possible adverse effects, and on economical choices as compared to other available options.

The 2009 Evidence-Based Clinical Practice Guidelines for Integrative Oncology: Complementary Therapies and Botanicals cover the following topics:

- Inquiry regarding CAM use.
- Offering guidance regarding CAM by a qualified professional.
- The use of CAM modalities to reduce specific symptoms.
- The role of regular physical activity in cancer care.
- The role of specific dietary supplements in cancer prevention.

- The role of nutritional supplements in cancer treatment.

In 2013, SIO published a review of the literature surrounding the treatment of lung cancer and the used of complementary therapies. Several complementary therapies may be helpful in improving the overall care of patients diagnosed with lung cancer. The evidenced-based clinical practice guidelines, Complementary Therapies and Integrative Medicine in Lung Cancer: Diagnosis and Management of Lung Cancer, are accessible free of charge here http://www.ncbi.nlm.nih.gov/pubmed/23649450

Deng, G. E., Rausch, S. M., Jones, L. W., Gulati, A., Kumar, N. B., Greenlee, H., . . . Cassileth, B. R. (2013). Complementary therapies and integrative medicine in lung cancer: Diagnosis and management of lung cancer, 3rd ed: American College of Chest Physicians evidence-based clinical practice guidelines. Chest, 143(5 Suppl), e420S-436S. doi: 10.1378/chest.12-2364.

Society of Integrative Oncology, 2009, Evidence-Based Clinical Practice Guidelines for Integrative Oncology: Complementary Therapies and Botanicals, http://www.integrativeonc.org/index.php/docguide

Three other health organizations, the National Cancer Institute, the National Center for Complementary and

Alternative Medicine, and the Oncology Nursing Society have a vested interest in cancer CAM.

THE NATIONAL CANCER INSTITUTE

The NCI has developed a series of peer-reviewed summaries of the latest information about the use of CAM in cancer care. As of this time, there are CAM PDQs in the following topic areas:

- CAM Therapies: 714-X, Acupuncture, Antineoplastons, Aromatherapy and Essential Oils, Cancelll/Cantron/Protocel, Cannais and Cannabinoids, Cartilage (Bovine and Shark), Coenzyme Q10, Essiac/Flor Essence, Gerson Therapy, Gonzalez Regimen, High-Dose Vitamin C, Hydrazine Sulfate, Laetrile/Amygdalin, Milk Thistle, Mistletoe Extract, Newcastle Disease Virus, PC-SPES, Selected Vegetables/Sun's Soup http://www.cancer.gov/cancertopics/pdq/cam
- CAM Topics: Prostate Cancer, Nutrition, and Dietary Supplements, Spirituality in Cancer Care, and CAM in Cancer Treatment
- Thinking about CAM: A Guide for People with Cancer http://www.cancer.gov/cancertopics/cam/thinking-about-CAM

National Center for Complementary and Alternative Medicine

NCCAM has a series of resources for consumers and health professionals in the area of cancer CAM to include specific modalities, clinical practice guidelines, and access to compiled systematic reviews and clinical studies.

General Information

- Antioxidants and Health: An Introduction http://nccam.nih.gov/health/antioxidants/introduction.htm
- Vitamin E Supplements http://nccam.nih.gov/news/alerts/vitamine/vitamine.htm
- Scientific literature updated continually on cancer CAM systematic reviews, clinical reviews, and meta-analyses in cancer CAM http://nccam.nih.gov/health/cancer (*see Scientific Literature section for link to current tab*)
- Cancer CAM clinical studies http://nccam.nih.gov/health/cancer (see Randomized Controlled Trials section for link to current tab)

Herbs at a Glance Series:

- Garlic http://nccam.nih.gov/health/garlic/ataglance.htm

- Green Tea http://nccam.nih.gov/health/greentea
- European Mistletoe http://nccam.nih.gov/health/mistletoe
- Soy http://nccam.nih.gov/health/soy/ataglance.htm

Clinical Practice Guidelines

- Vitamin, Mineral, and Multivitamin Supplements for the Primary Prevention of Cardiovascular Disease and Cancer http://www.uspreventiveservicestaskforce.org/uspstf14/vitasupp/vitasuppfinalrs.htm
- American Cancer Society Guidelines on Nutrition and Physical Activity for Cancer Prevention http://onlinelibrary.wiley.com/doi/10.3322/caac.20140/pdf
- American College of Sports Medicine Roundtable on Exercise Guidelines for Cancer Survivors http://journals.lww.com/acsm-msse/Fulltext/2010/07000/American_College_of_Sports_Medicine_Roundtable_on.23.aspx

Oncology Nursing Society

In 2009, The Oncology Nursing Society published an updated version to their position paper on the use of complementary, alternative, and integrative therapies in cancer care. Oncology nurses provide care for individuals with cancer often without knowledge of their CAM use. ONS and its affiliates promote funding and collaboration in the design of methodologically rigorous supportive care and treatment studies involving CAM therapies.

Oncology nurses are encouraged to:

- Evaluate their personal and professional beliefs regarding CAM use
- Assess and document CAM use among patients with cancer
- Seek training and credentialing if practicing CAM therapies
- Develop a working knowledge of CAM-related issues such as reimbursement, liability, and ethical/legal topics

Oncology Nursing Society, 2009, Position: The Use of Complementary, Alternative, and Integrative Therapies in Cancer Care, http://www2.ons.org/Publications/Positions/media/ons/docs/positions/alternativetherapies.pdf

§

Resources

Handbook on Integrative Oncology Nursing (2010, Decker, G., Lee, C [this book author]).

This new guide defines complementary and alternative medicine (CAM), examines the issue of making

*integrative assessments, identifies commonly used thera-
pies, and takes a close look at how symptoms can be man-
aged using CAM therapies.*

*Symptoms representing a wide range including
Anorexia-Cachexia Syndrome, Cognitive Dysfunction,
Constipation, Depression, Diarrhea, Fatigue,
Hormonal Changes and Hot Flashes, Insomnia,
Mucositis, Myelosuppression, Nausea and Vomiting,
Sexuality Alterations, Taste Changes, and Xerostomia
are covered in this book.*

Cancer and Complementary Medicine: Your Guide to
Smart Choices in Symptom Management (2012, Lee, C
[this book author], Decker, G.)

*This new guide provides an introduction to CAM and
its use in cancer symptom management, allowing patients to make informed and safe choices. Chapters ex-
amine issues such as symptom management, healthy
living, safe usage of CAM, and types of CAM available
as well as detailed information on herbs, vitamins, and
supplements.*

17

Cancer Care Systems: Role of Preventative Medicine

What have we covered so far?

Thus far, we have covered the foundational components of cancer care, symptom management, integrative oncology, guideline development, screening and treatment guidelines.

In the next five chapters, the cancer care system is discussed from several viewpoints: the role of preventative medicine, impact of sustained interest in cancer screening, the role of shared and informed decision making in conversations about cancer, the role of the human genome, and how/where these pieces all come together in the age of personalized and precise medicine.

What is preventative medicine?

Prevention is an action taken to decrease the chance of getting a disease or condition. As an example, cancer prevention includes avoiding risk factors and increasing protective factors (see chapter 1 for cancer risk factors).

Preventative medicine is the anticipation and offsetting of disease or injury in individuals and populations (Tabers, 2014).

Three types of cancer prevention exist: primary, secondary, and tertiary with examples given as seen in **Table 25**.

Table 25. Primary, Secondary, and Tertiary Prevention Defined with Examples		
Category of Prevention	*Definition*	*Example(s) in Cancer Care*
Primary	The prevention of a cancer from ever developing or to delay its development.	Prophylactic surgery to prevent or reduce the risk of developing a malignancy.
Secondary	The identification of individuals who are at risk for developing cancer and starting screening tests based on the risk assessment.	Use of the Pap smear to detect cervical cancer, mammography to detect breast cancer, or colonoscopy to remove a polyp or colon cancer.
Tertiary	The monitoring for and preventing recurrence of a diagnosed cancer; screening for second primary cancers and long-term effects of treatment in cancer survivors	Detecting complications and second cancers in long-term survivors.

How can preventative medicine rise to a level of necessary importance in health care today?

In the past, the field of medicine focused on developing new treatments, new devices, and new procedures for disease management. Preventative science, learning the causes and prevention of diseases in individuals and populations, has been less of a priority as compared to treatment. Health officials agree that attention to prevention can potentially lead to overall better individual health, national health and world-wide health.

> *"Investing in prevention should be a strategic national priority to help improve the lagging population health of the United States compared with peer countries." (Yach & Calitz 2014, p 791).*

Are there federal and private sector resources dedicated to preventative medicine and research?

The NIH Office of Disease Prevention (ODP) is in charge of assessing, facilitating, and stimulating research in health promotion and disease prevention and sharing research results to improve public health of the nation. The prevention of disease is superior to treatment, and the knowledge gained from this research leads to rigorous clinical practice, health policy, and community health programs. The NIH-ODP identified 6 priorities to improve prevention research within the agency and nation:

- Identify research areas efforts.
- Monitor research efforts and assess the progress and results of research.
- Promote best available research methods.
- Promote collaborative projects across the NIH, the public and private entities.
- Promote evidence-based interventions and sharing of research in prevention.
- Increase the visibility of this research at the NIH and across the country.

In the private sector, an example of one effort promote preventative medicine is in software development. Major technology companies are designing personally-intelligent devices to monitor health behavior.

Yach and Calitz (2014) support efforts geared toward prevention science in the US with the following actions:

- Increase research on non-communicable diseases in community settings.
- Ensure that NIH institutes increase their support for prevention science.

- Encourage the NIH foundation to continue to develop public-private partnerships focused on prevention science.
- Ensure that the personalized health technology models endorsed by the National Human Genome Research Institute (http://www.genome.gov/ELSI/) are also supporting basic and applied research in the area.

Finally, legislation exists through the Affordable Care Act (ACA) assuring that most health plans cover a set of preventive services. Examples of preventative services in the oncology population are colorectal cancer screening, HPV injections, and tobacco use screening (Healthcare.gov, 2014).

§

References

Oncology Nursing Society, Types of Prevention: http://www2.ons.org/ClinicalResources/BreastCancer/Prevention/Types

Tabers (2014). Preventative Medicine. http://www.tabers.com/tabersonline/view/Tabers-Dictionary/768227/all/medicine?q=personalized%20medicine#58

Yach, D. and C. Calitz (2014). "New opportunities in the changing landscape of prevention." JAMA 312(8): 791-792.

18

Cancer Care Systems: Sustained Interest in Screening

In proportion to its earnings, the US spends more money on health care than any other nation in the world (IOM, 2012). With the increases in cancer detection through screening, the number of cancer survivors has increased in the past several decades to more than 13 million. The number of survivors is estimated to reach 18 million by the year 2022. (McCabe, et al 2013, Siegel, et al, 2012).

Is there a continued interest in cancer screening in the US?

Despite the potential for false positives and use of unproven screening tests, the answer is <u>yes</u>. Most individuals in the US are committed to cancer screening. In order to quantify the level of interest in cancer screening, researchers conducted a telephone survey of 500 men age 50 and order and women aged 40 and older without a history of cancer between 2001 and 2002 (Schwartz, et. al 2004). The results were:

Regarding Cancer Screening:

- Cancer screening is "almost always a good idea" according to 87% of the adults surveyed.
- Cancer screening saves lives "most" or "all of the time" according to 74% of the adults surveyed.
- Cancer screening usually reduces the amount of necessary treatment when cancer is detected according to 53% of the adults surveyed.
- Individuals (66%) wanted to be tested for cancer even if there was no treatment available.
- Individuals (56%) wanted to be tested for slow growing cancers that even untreated would not ever cause clinical problems.
- Individuals (64%) believed there are "about the right number" of screening tests available.

Regarding Personal Commitment to Cancer Screening:

- Most adults (99%) have had cancer screening such as Papanicolaou testing, mammograms, PSA test, sigmoidoscopy or colonoscopy.

- Women (58%) would overrule their physician if he/she suggested less frequent Papanicolaou testing.
- Men (77%) would overrule their physician if he/she suggested less frequent PSA testing.
- Men and women (74%) would continue would overrule their physician if he/she suggested less often colon cancer screening.

Regarding Screening as Obligatory in Health Care

- Given a scenario of a 55-year old woman in average health foregoing Papanicolaou testing, individuals (79%) believed that this was "irresponsible."
- Given a scenario of a 55-year old man or woman in average health foregoing colonoscopy, individuals (54%) believed that this was "irresponsible."
- Given a scenario of an 80-year old woman in average health foregoing mammography, individuals (41%) believed that this was "irresponsible."
- Given a scenario of an 80-year old man or woman in average health foregoing colonoscopy, individuals (32%) believed that this was "irresponsible."

IS THERE A DOWN-SIDE TO THE INTERPRETATION OF THIS DATA?

Despite the systematic manner in which the data was gathered and the information it provides to our understanding of some beliefs regarding screening, the answer is yes. The reasons are:

- The study respondents were limited to those with telephones, and some populations may have been under-represented.
- The study does not speak to the specific reasons *why* individuals are interested in screening.
- Screening campaigns using phrases that imply a sense of duty or responsibility to undergo cancer screening may bias the public against personal "choice."
- The belief that "relief" when a test result is wrong (a false-positive; cancer is not present) outweighs "fear" that it might be right (cancer is present).

This 2004 survey was the first to systematically assess and circulate data regarding public interest in cancer screening. Given the increase in media attention, medical information on the internet, and high-profile individuals' support of cancer screening over the past decade, it may be valuable to compare the results of this survey, replicating the original design, with similar data in real time. Additionally, continued screening in the US will require collaboration and synchronicity between key health stakeholders who are simultaneously adapting to frequent changes in the economy and health care trends.

§

References

McCabe, M., Bhatia, Sm., Oeffinger, K., Reaman, G., Tyne, C., Wollins, D., Hudson, M. (2013). American Society of Clinical Oncology Statement: Achieving high-Quality Cancer Survivorship Care, Journal of Clinical Oncology, 31(5), 631-640.

Siegel, R., et al. (2012). "Cancer treatment and survivorship statistics, 2012." CA Cancer J Clin 62(4): 220-241.

Schwartz, L. M., Woloshin, S., Fowler, F. J., Jr., & Welch, H. G. (2004). Enthusiasm for cancer screening in the United States. JAMA, 291(1), 71-78. doi: 10.1001/jama.291.1.71

19

Cancer Care Systems: Informed and Shared Decision Making

What are the benefits of patient involvement in their health care decision making?

Patient involvement in health care decision making has grown from a general interest on behalf of patients to a near necessity in assuring the best overall outcomes to meet patient's needs. Partnering between patients and providers to form a "patient-provider partnership" is necessary to be sure that patients' wants, needs, and preferences are upheld. Additionally, these partnerships are necessary to ensure patients are educated and receive needed support required to make informed decisions and participate fully in their own health care.

The specific benefits of patient involvement are:

- Patient autonomy
- Independent and rational decision-making
- Trust in the patient-provider partnership
- Confidence in participation in care
- Knowledge about screening options
- Realistic expectations about benefits/harms

WHAT IS INFORMED DECISION MAKING AND SHARED DECISION MAKING?

In the early 2000s, the concepts of 'informed decision making' and 'shared decision making' first became commonplace in the literature. These concepts build upon one another. First, informed decision making describes a process in which an patient gathers information from clinicians and other clinical/nonclinical source *with or without* either party weighing in on beliefs/values regarding the information during the information-gathering process.

Second, shared decision making describes a process in which both the patient and the clinician share information *with one another*, agree *with one another* on a course of action, and take steps to jointly participate in the decision-making process. This process takes into account that the patient understands the risks of the condition, the treatment alternatives, weighs his/her values with the benefits/harms of the intervention(s), and participates in the decision-making process at a level that he/she feels comfortable (Sheridan, et. al, 2004; Kaplan, 2004).

When the USPSTF report on shared decision making was published in 2004, there was vagueness surrounding the relationship between shared decision making and improvement in overall health outcomes. At that time, evidence that shared decision making improved health outcomes was described as "indirect and mixed" (Sheridan, et. al., 2004, p. 60).

Patient variables were:

- Ability to gather reliable information
- Ability to convey thoughts/beliefs regarding gathered information
- Ability to understand medical concepts
- Age and/or education level
- Understanding that medicine is not an 'exact science'
- Lack of understanding that a decision was needed
- Discomfort in the decision-making process
- Ethnicity and potential impact on health care beliefs
- Fear and/or regret that decisions that may turn out poorly

WHAT ARE THE BARRIERS TO CLINICIANS ALLOWING PATIENT INVOLVEMENT IN HEALTH CARE DECISION MAKING?

In order for patients to fully engage in shared decision making, clinicians may need to consider their own concerns and misconceptions regarding patient participation. Interest on behalf of clinicians to engage in this joint process is vital, but there may be real or perceived barriers to the process.

Clinician variables include:

- Lack of time in scheduled visits
- Lack of financial reimbursement in discussing screening options
- Lack of training in interviewing techniques needed to engage patients in shared decision making
- Lack of evidence about benefits/harms of screening interventions coupled with inability to communicate technical aspects of the tests in plain language.

IS PATIENT INVOLVEMENT IN SHARED DECISION MAKING "ALL OR NONE?"

Patient involvement in shared decision making is not "all or none" in terms of the spectrum extending from "all" on one end to "none" on the other end. One end of the spectrum is the where the patient must be knowledgeable about every aspect of every decision, fully understand all the medical facets, and in complete control in every facet of decision-making process. The other end of the spectrum is where the patient does not require knowledge, understanding, or inclusion in the decision-making process. The USPSTF asserted that although shared decision making may be ideal, patient participation is considered satisfactory when the patient feels comfortable.

HOW CAN CLINICIANS FACILITATE SHARING DECISION MAKING?

In five-steps, the USPSTF outlined an approach to shared decision making:

1. Assess the patient's health needs and desired role in decision making.
2. Advise the patient regarding screening options and provide evidence-based information about the benefits/harms/alternatives/scientific uncertainties.
3. Agree to discuss the patient's values, determine patient preferences, and mutually decide a course of action.
4. Assist with the delivery or prescribing of the screening option.
5. Arrange for a follow-up discussion of the plan

§

COLLEEN O. LEE

References

Kaplan, R. M. (2004). Shared medical decision making: A new tool for preventive medicine. Am J Prev Med, 26(1), 81-83. doi: http://dx.doi.org/10.1016/j.amepre.2003.09.022

Sheridan, S. L., Harris, R. P., & Woolf, S. H. (2004). Shared decision making about screening and chemoprevention. a suggested approach from the U.S. Preventive Services Task Force. Am J Prev Med, 26(1), 56-

20

Genetics:
DNA, DNA Sequencing, and the Human Genome Project

What is a gene?

Deoxyribonucleic acid (DNA) is the chemical compound that holds the "instructions" required to develop and direct the actions of nearly all living organisms. DNA molecules are made of two twisted, paired strands, often referred to as a "double helix." Each single DNA strand is made of four chemicals, called nucleotide bases, which consist of the genetic "alphabet."

The bases are

- adenine (A)
- thymine (T)
- guanine (G)
- cytosine (C).

Bases on the other single strand are also present. The bases "pair" specifically, for example, an A always pairs with a T; a C always pairs with a G. The order of the bases, A, T, C and G, determines the information in that part of the DNA molecule. A living organism's complete set of DNA is called its "genome." Nearly every single cell in the body contains a complete set of the approximately 3 billion DNA base pairs hat make up the human genome. With its four-letter set, DNA contains the information needed to build the entire human body.

A gene is a unit of DNA that carries the information for making a protein molecule or set of protein molecules. Each of the nearly 20,000 to 25,000 genes in the human genome "codes" for about three proteins. These proteins make up organs and tissues in the body, as well as regulate chemical reactions and carry signals between cells. If a cell's DNA is changed or mutated, an abnormal protein may form. This abnormal protein can disrupt the body's normal processes and lead to a disease such as cancer.

WHAT IS DNA SEQUENCING?
DNA "sequencing" is systematically defining the exact order of the bases in a strand of DNA. The most common type of sequencing used today is called 'sequencing by synthesis' where DNA polymerase (the enzyme in cells that makes DNA) is used to make a new strand of DNA from a particular

strand of interest. This method can generate 'reads' of 125 base pairs in a row and billions of 'reads' at a time.

Researchers can use DNA sequencing to search for mutations that may play a role in the development or advancement of a disease. The mutation may be a substitution, deletion, or addition of a single base pair or a deletion of thousands of bases.

The Human Genome Project, led by the National Human Genome Research Institute (NHGRI) at the NIH, formed a very high-quality, free version of the human genome sequence available in public databases as of April 2003. The sequence is a composite from nearly 100 individuals. The Project was designed to generate a resource that could be used to look for the genetic mutations that increase risk of specific diseases (such as cancer) or to look for the type of genetic mutations frequently seen in cancerous cells. Future research projects can then understand how the genome functions and to discover the genetic basis for living organisms' health and disease. (NHGRI, 2014).

How does the Human Genome Project impact our health now?

Nearly every human disease or condition has some basis in our genes. With the DNA data made available by the Human Genome Project and other genome-based (genomic) research, scientists and clinicians have more available tools to study the role that genetics plays in the disease process. These diseases (e.g. cancer, diabetes, and heart disease) create the majority of health problems in the US. Genomic research is already helping researchers to develop better diagnostic tools, more effective treatments, and evidence-based approaches for patients and providers.

A key facet is that it frequently takes time, effort, and funding to move discoveries from the laboratory into the clinic (also known as 'bench to bedside'). Most new treatments in the form of drugs that are based on genome-based research at least 10 to 15 years away. Generally, it may take more than a decade for a commercial company to perform the types of clinical studies necessary to receive approval from the Food and Drug Administration.

The cost of sequencing the Human Genome has decreased exponentially over the past decades, beginning in the late 1990s at about 3 billion dollars to possibly a little less than 1000 dollars in the near future. Ultimately, it appears that future treatments in the US will be tailored to a patient's specific genomic makeup. **Table 26** outlines the declining costs of sequencing the genome.

Table 26. Declining Cost of Sequencing the Human Genome	
Year	Cost in dollars
Late 1990s	3 billion
2001	100-300 million
2007	10 million
2009	50,000
2011	5000
2014-2015	Nearing 1000 or less

Wetterstrand KA. DNA Sequencing Costs: Data from the NHGRI Genome Sequencing Program (GSP) Available at: www.genome.gov/sequencingcosts

Robson (2014) addresses the future potential for affordable sequencing genes as the first step toward a "comprehensive genomic medicine paradigm" in the US. This level of precision and knowledge can and will impact primary care and most significantly, cancer care. The combined efforts of the cancer care team, including nurses, oncologists, genetic counselors, and cancer geneticists are needed to 'drive the paradigm shift' toward personalized or precision medicine and to ensure the inclusion of 'next generation' technology into the practice of preventive medicine and preventative oncology.

§

REFERENCES

Kurian, A. W., et al. (2014). "Clinical evaluation of a multiple-gene sequencing panel for hereditary cancer risk assessment." J Clin Oncol 32(19): 2001-2009.

Robson, M. (2014). "Multigene panel testing: planning the next generation of research studies in clinical cancer genetics." J Clin Oncol 32(19): 1987-1989.

Stadler, Z. K., et al. (2014). "Cancer genomics and inherited risk." J Clin Oncol 32(7): 687-698.

21

CANCER CARE SYSTEMS: PERSONALIZED AND PRECISE MEDICINE

WHAT IS PERSONALIZED MEDICINE?

The term 'personalized medicine' is defined narrowly and broadly depending on the context in which it is discussed. The general concept, developed centuries ago, involves the inquiry into individual characteristics thought to impact development and/or response to diseases or medical conditions. Scientists and researchers have studied and continue to study why different individuals experience disease or respond to treatment differently. When the characteristics of a disease or condition are identified, preventive or treatment interventions can then focus on those who will benefit, thereby sparing the expense and side effects for those who will not. **Table 27** lists various definitions for personalized and precision medicine.

Table 27. Personalized and/or Precision Medicine Range of Definitions	
Source	*Definition*
FDA	The tailoring of treatment to the individual characteristics, needs, and preferences of a patient during all stages of care, including prevention, diagnosis, treatment, and follow-up.
National Academy of Sciences	The tailoring of treatment to the individual characteristics of each patient and the ability to classify individuals into subpopulations that vary in the biology, susceptibility, and/or response to a particular disease. It does <u>not</u> mean the development of drugs or devices that are unique to a patient.
National Institutes of Health	The use of an individual's genetic profile to guide decisions surrounding the prevention, diagnosis, and treatment of disease. Knowledge of a patient's genetic profile aids in the selection of the proper medication or therapy and administration of the proper dose or regimen.
Personalized Medicine Coalition	A multi-faceted approach to patient care that improves the ability to diagnose and treat disease plus offer the potential to detect disease at an earlier stage when it is easier to treat effectively. The full implementation of personalized medicine encompasses: risk assessment, prevention, detection, diagnosis, treatment, and management.
Taber's Online Medical Dictionary	The study of an individual's unique biochemical and genetic makeup in order to determine the susceptibility to disease or potential responses to treatment.

Personalized medicine has also been termed any of the following depending on how the term is used in context:

- Precision medicine
- Stratified medicine
- Targeted medicine
- Pharmacogenomics

The field of pharmacogenetics factors in the involvement of genes in an individual's response to medications.

In doing this, it covers basic drug development research, pharmacokinetics [how and the rate to which drugs are metabolized], patient genetic testing and clinical patient management. The goal of pharmacogenetics is to predict a patient's genetic response to a specific medication as a means of delivering the best treatment. By predicting the drug response of an individual, it will be possible to increase a therapies' success and decrease the rate of adverse side effects.

In their frequently-cited 2001 article on pharmacogenetics, Spear, Heath-Chiozzi and Huff presented the response rates of patients to drug therapy for several major medical conditions (see **Table 28**). Individuals with cancer were anticipated to have approximately a 25% response rate to the chemotherapy drugs they were given for the treatment of their disease. While it is important to note that lack of drug efficacy in a given patient reflects many factors [drug-related factors (inadequate or inaccurate dosing) or patient-related factors (lack of adherence)], the end result of a 25% response rate is not sufficient to treat a serious disease such as cancer.

Table 28. Response Rates of Drug Therapy for Selected Medical Conditions (≤50%)	
Condition	*Response Rate*
Cancer	25%
Alzheimer's Disease	30%
Osteoporosis	48%
Migraines (prevention)	50%
Rheumatoid Arthritis	50%

For a drug to be approved for use in humans, it must be safe and effective. This safety and efficacy evaluation is completed through clinical trials within particular patient populations. It is rare for a drug to be safe or effective for everyone (Spear, Heath-Chiozzi and Huff, 2001). The variability among individuals has a significant effect on the quality and cost of healthcare, and in this realm, cancer care.

What are companion diagnostics?

Device manufacturers work directly with the FDA to develop and refine aids to diagnose specific cancer genetic mutations. These aids, termed companion diagnostics, are medical devices that assist oncology providers in determining which treatments to offer and which doses to prescribe all tailored directly to the patient. Companion diagnostics can show not only which patients could be helped by a drug but also which patients would *not* benefit.

There are currently 19 FDA approved/cleared companion diagnostic tests for the selection of drug to treat various disease and conditions. The specific cancer-related tests are listed in **Appendix A4**.

§

References

Food and Drug Administration http://www.fda.gov/ScienceResearch/SpecialTopics/PersonalizedMedicine/default.htm

Institute of Medicine, (2013), Delivering High-Quality Cancer Care Questions for Patients with Cancer to Ask Their Care Team, http://www.iom.edu/~/media/Files/Report%20Files/2013/Quality-Cancer-Care/qualitycan-cercare_insert2.pdf

National Academy of Science (2011) Toward Precision Medicine: Building a Knowledge Network for Biomedical Research and a New Taxonomy of Disease, http://www.nap.edu/download.php?record_id=13284

NIH http://www.tabers.com/tabersonline/view/Tabers-Dictionary/768227/all/medicine?q=personalized%20medicine#58

Paving the Way for Personalized Medicine, October 2013, http://www.fda.gov/downloads/ScienceResearch/SpecialTopics/PersonalizedMedicine/UCM372421.pdf

Personalized Medicine Coalition, The Age of Personalized Medicine (2009), http://personalizedmedicinecoalition. org/Userfiles/PMC-Corporate/file/pmc_age_of_pmc_factsheet.pdf

Spear, B. B., et al. (2001). "Clinical application of pharmacogenetics." Trends Mol Med 7(5): 201-204.

Tabers: http://www.tabers.com/tabersonline/view/Tabers-Dictionary/768227/all/medicine?q=personalized%20medicine#58

22

Cancer Care Systems: Delivering Care with the Highest Quality

How has cancer care improved in the past decade?

In the last section, we reviewed the history behind shared decision making in health care and the barriers on behalf of patients and clinicians. This brand-new work advanced the efforts of patients everywhere to have a voice in their care and have their voice be supported by the medical community. While patient participation in decision making today in real time remains largely unquantified and the "all or none" spectrum of patient involvement in decision making still exits, the gaps are not as wide as they were a decade ago.

Cancer care has improved over the past decade in many areas. Advances specifically in detection, prevention, and treatment between 1999 to 2008 include the following progress:

- Gradually falling death rates from *all* cancers
- Gradually falling death rates for *most* cancer sites including the four most common cancers: lung, colorectal, breast, and prostate. (Eheman, et. al, 2012).

In an effort to promote continued advances in cancer care, the Institute of Medicine (IOM) National Cancer Policy Forum convened a public workshop in 2012 named *Delivering Affordable Cancer Care in the 21st Century* to address these and other topics.

WHAT WERE THE PROPOSED SUGGESTIONS TO IMPROVE THE AFFORDABILITY AND QUALITY OF CANCER CARE?

The 2012 IOM workshop participants offered suggestions and possible solutions to improve affordability and quality in cancer care which included the following:

- Improve the quality of available cancer-related information so patients can make decisions and manage their care.
- Encourage clinicians to provide affordable, high-quality cancer care.
- Uphold and assist with best practices in cancer care
- Increase research that advises clinical practice.

- Build in rewards for the delivery of affordable, high-quality cancer care by improvements in reimbursement and delivery systems.

Table 29 outlines each of these proposed suggestions with examples of how best to implement them.

Table 29. Suggestions and Solutions to Improve Affordability and Quality of Cancer Care (IOM 2012)		
Suggestion/Solution		*Examples*
1. Improve the quality of available cancer-related information so patients can make decisions and manage their care	a.	Assist patients in selecting clinicians by providing quality of care criteria
	b.	Reimburse clinicians for time spent communicating with patients regarding cancer diagnosis, cost of care, treatment benefits/harms, palliative care, and hospice care
2. Encourage clinicians to provide affordable, high-quality cancer care	a.	Ensure that clinicians are trained to analyze study findings, understand cost considerations of various treatment options, and communicate this information well to patients
	b.	Encourage clinicians to not suggest treatment options with uncertain/questionable value
	c.	Encourage clinicians to adhere to the American Society for Clinical Oncology "top five" list of opportunities to improve quality and value in cancer care (http://www.asco.org/press-center/asco-publishes-top-five-list-opportunities-improve-quality-and-value-cancer-care)
	d.	Include cost considerations in clinical practice guidelines and treatment pathways
3. Uphold and assist with best practices in cancer care	a.	Support care models (e.g. team-based) that provide 24-hour support to patients
	b.	Ensure initiation of palliative and hospice care earlier in the cancer care delivery model
	c.	Improve the use of and ability for interaction in electronic medical record systems
	d.	Provide available information to patients, clinicians, and payers about cancer care (quality of care, outcomes, cost) in various populations
4. Increase research that advises clinical practice	a.	Develop learning systems that gather data on health care topics to assist in decision making in personalized medicine, research approaches, redesigning health care, and quality cancer care
	b.	Sponsor clinical studies involving real time comparisons among specific patient populations
5. Build in rewards for the delivery of affordable, high-quality cancer care by improvements in reimbursement and delivery systems	a.	Reimburse clinicians for performance on patient-provider communication
	b.	Support programs to assess new/novel advances in cancer care
	c.	Reduce/eliminate the connection between treatment options and provider income
	d.	Review/evaluate cancer care delivery systems such as medical homes and shared savings programs
	e.	Redesign payment options to encourage patient use of higher-value treatment options instead of lower-value treatment options

ARE THERE CURRENT EFFORTS UNDERWAY TO UNDERSTAND CANCER CARE IN REAL TIME?

Recognizing the persistent gaps in cancer care and unanticipated new opportunities that arise, high-quality cancer care remains a goal not yet widely achieved. In the face of these gaps and opportunities, the cost of cancer care is universally rising at a faster rate as compared to other diseases (IOM, 2013). The Committee on Improving the Quality of Cancer Care convened again to address the gaps and opportunities, acknowledging,

> *"In many ways, oncology care is an extreme example of the best and worst in the health care system today— highly innovative targeted diagnostics and therapeutics alongside escalating costs that do not consistently relate to the clinical value of treatments, tremendous waste and inefficiencies due to poor coordination of care, and lack of adherence to evidence-based guidelines with frequent use of ineffective or inappropriate treatments "* *(IOM, 2013, Patricia Ganz, p. xvi).*

To plan a new pathway for the delivery of high-quality cancer care, the crisis needs to be explained:

- The number of older adults will double between 2010 and 2030 in the US. This doubling will lead to a 30% increase in the number of cancer survivors and a 45% increase in the incidence of cancer.

- The number of health care personnel assisting individuals with cancer is decreasing leading to gaps in quality care. Training programs are unable to provide adequate training leaving family and direct care givers to provide care without suitable support or guidance.
- The cost of cancer care has increased from $72 billion dollars in 2004 to $125 billion in 2010. Increased costs are anticipate to rise another 39% to $173 billion dollars by 2020.
- New available knowledge in the field requires clinicians to remain current and understand this information in order to treat various cancers accurately.
- Newly-developed tools designed to improve the quality of care, such as metrics, guidelines, and computer technology, are not yet widely available and have drawbacks.

Now recognizing the crisis, the IOM team developed six facets to a high-quality cancer care necessary to address the current crisis and offset the future crisis (IOM, 2013).

THE SIX FACETS ARE:

1. Patient engagement.
2. Trained workforce.
3. Evidence-based care.

4. Computer systems specific to cancer care.
5. Translation of evidence into clinical care, quality measures, and performance improvement.
6. Affordable and accessible cancer care.

WHAT ARE THE COMMON CONCEPTS IMPACTING THESE SIX FACETS?

- Direct to consumer marketing.
- Full transparency to patients.
- Commitment to share findings broadly.
- Robust engagement of patients in the research process.
- Thoughtful consideration about cancer screening decisions.
- Need for balanced and accurate information about the benefits and harms of cancer screening tests.
- Support for cancer screening tests should be to in-form decision-making.

WHAT QUESTIONS SHOULD PATIENTS ASK THEIR HEALTH CARE PROVIDERS?

The IOM developed a succinct guide of helpful questions for patients to ask their providers. This guide focuses on prognosis, treatment, advance care planning, and family/psychosocial/spiritual needs (IOM, 2013).

- The questions surrounding <u>prognosis</u> are geared toward knowing the goal of treatment, life expectancy, likelihood of a cure, options for care if treatment is not selected, when should hospice and/or palliative care be discussed?
- The questions surrounding <u>treatment</u> are geared toward knowing treatment options, risks/benefits of treatment, cost of treatment, eligibility for clinical trials, where to be treated, coordination of care, among others.
- The questions surrounding <u>advance care planning</u> are geared toward knowing who is involved in this level of planning, who can/should make decision in the event that the patient cannot, and what are the important legal/financial issues to discuss?
- The questions surrounding <u>family/psychosocial, and spiritual needs</u> are geared toward information-sharing with family and what resources are available to work through the complexities of cancer care?

What is the state of cancer care in America now?

The American Society for Clinical Oncology (ASCO) published the first annual report on the state of cancer care in the US. The report is in response to the IOM's 2013 *Delivering High Quality Cancer Care – Charting a*

New Course for a System in Crisis. By taking ASCO's proposed steps, the oncology community can move beyond 'crisis mode' to attain a cancer care system that promotes progress and delivers patient-centered, high-value care for cancer patients. Topics covered and recommendations are listed in ASCO's report are listed in **Table 30**.

Table 30. ASCO State of Cancer Care 2014 Topics and Recommendations	
Topic	*Recommendation*
Oncology Workforce	Ensure continued availability of oncologist services for patients nationwide. • Coordinate care with primary care providers. • Include telemedicine and visiting consultants • Monitor and treat oncologist burnout. • Promote diversity in oncology workforce.
State of Oncology Practice	Sustain oncology practices' ability to meet patient needs in every community. • Support struggling practices financially. • Test new cancer care delivery models. • Improve care reimbursement dollars.
Quality in Cancer Care	Enhance quality and consistency of care. • Develop national quality care systems. • Advance ASCO's CancerLinQ system. • Remove cancer health disparities in access to care. • Develop common measures of cancer care to better assess value.

WHAT ARE THE CRUCIAL CONCEPTS FOR CONSIDERATION FOR PATIENTS, FAMILY MEMBERS, AND THE GENERAL PUBLIC?

- Prevention of disease is superior to treatment.
- Gaps in cancer care exist.
- The number of older adults will double between 2010 and 2030 in the US.
- The number of clinicians assisting individuals and families with cancer is decreasing.
- The cost of cancer care is rising.
- Evidence-based guidelines are not in one place and not widely adopted.
- Shared decision making improves overall cancer care.
- High-quality cancer care remains a goal not yet widely achieved.
- New knowledge requires clinicians to remain current and understand this information in order to diagnose and treat different cancers precisely.
- New tools to improve the quality of care (technology, metrics, among others) are not yet widely available.

§

References

American Society for Clinical Oncology (ASCO, 2014). http://www.asco.org/sites/www.asco.org/files/cancerinamerica2014-lowres_1.pdf

Eheman, C., Henley, S. J., Ballard-Barbash, R., Jacobs, E. J., Schymura, M. J., Noone, A. M., . . . Edwards, B. K. (2012). Annual Report to the Nation on the status of cancer, 1975-2008, featuring cancers associated with excess weight and lack of sufficient physical activity. Cancer, 118(9), 2338-2366. doi: 10.1002/cncr.27514

Institute of Medicine (2013), Delivering High Quality Cancer Care – Charting a New Course for a System in Crisis, http://www.iom.edu/Reports/2013/Delivering-High-Quality-Cancer-Care-Charting-a-New-Course-for-a-System-in-Crisis.aspx

23

PERSONALIZED MEDICINE AND YOU

WHAT HAVE WE COVERED SO FAR?

Thus far, we have covered the foundational components of cancer care, symptom management, integrative oncology, guideline development, screening and treatment guidelines, the role of preventative medicine, impact of sustained interest in cancer screening, the role of shared and informed decision making, the human genome, and how/where these pieces all come together in the age of personalized and precise medicine. The general public and healthcare providers are inundated with new information involving how to monitor and improve our health. In terms of cancer prevention, and for some, cancer treatment and survivorship, the puzzle pieces are many and often overwhelming in number.

How can we put the puzzle pieces together in cancer care today to personalize medicine for our generation?

Education

The first step is education. In this electronic age, access to quality cancer-related healthcare information is available on the internet, if not in the home, then in the local library. And libraries (public or in a hospital) are a good source for both printed and electronic information. Librarians can assist with electronic searches and book stack literature.

- For those with a strong family history of cancer, learn about the risk factors and preventative measures.
- For those with cancer, use the resources listed in Appendix A6 as a starting point in learning about the diagnosis, treatment, supportive care, and survivorship considerations.
- Carefully listen to medical news reports for information on:
  - ✓ Who sponsored the study and who is reporting the results.
  - ✓ Independent analysis of study design and results.

✓ Evidence of publication in peer-reviewed forums.
✓ Recognition of study limitations and sample sizes.
✓ The 'price tag' on new technology in light of its overall benefit in prevention, diagnosis, or treatment of the medical condition.

COMMUNICATION

The second step is communication with your healthcare providers. Talk openly about appropriate cancer screening based on age and gender.

- For those with a strong family history of cancer, this conversation can happen yearly and whenever there is a change in providers.
- For those with cancer, keep a log of the events and an ongoing list of questions about your diagnosis, treatment, supportive care, and survivorship considerations. One of the greatest gaps in cancer care is communication between providers. Keep your oncology team connected with your primary healthcare team. Make routine office visits with your primary provider while you are going through cancer treatment and recovery. Arrange for the sending of your medical records from your cancer treatment visits to your primary provider.

- Think about the level of involvement you would like in your healthcare decisions and make this known. For example, be clear about how you would like to hear information whether good or bad and who you would like to have with you during this information exchange.

Planning

The third step is planning your healthcare. Plan to access preventative and routine healthcare services, monitor the results, and keep a personal file of your healthcare information (lab values, medication list, reports of testing in a chronological order) with reminders for next appointments. Routine appointments such as eye care and dental care, and can be scheduled well in advance to assure adherence.

Supporters of personalized medicine foresee a time in the future where individuals have their genome sequencing linked to the medical record. This would allow health care providers to develop a proactive strategy based on potential susceptibility to diseases and conditions with an anticipated response to various types of medication. While the healthcare and medical-legal infrastructure has not been developed yet to support this effort, its reality is approaching sooner given the decreasing cost of sequencing over the past decade. Paving the pathway for this upcoming change in the way our health is viewed and catalogued will require individual and corporate planning.

- For those individuals who will have their genome sequenced, plan on how/where that information will be used, shared, and saved confidentially.
- Using the guide in Table 31, plan out your cancer screening for yourself and your loved ones if you and your healthcare provider determine that you are at average risk for cancer.
- After the age of 70 years, individuals should discuss their screening activities specifically with their provider. Routine cancer screening in this age groups has implications on healthcare resources and possible unnecessary procedures and overtreatment (Royce, Hendrix, Stokes, Allen, & Chen, 2014).

Table 31. Age-related Cancer Screening Recommendations for the General Population (Average Risk) for Breast, Cervical, Colorectal, Lung, and Prostate Cancers

Age	Men	Women
20-30		Breast self-exam, Clinical breast exam every 3 years; Pap Test every 3 years
30-40		Breast self-exam, Clinical breast exam every 3 years; Pap Test and HPV test every 3-5 years (discuss with provider)
40-50		Breast self-exam, Clinical breast exam yearly, Screening mammography (discuss with provider); Pap Test and HPV test every 3-5 years (discuss with provider)
50-60	Colonoscopy every 10 years; flexible sigmoidoscopy or virtual colonoscopy every 5 years; PSA blood test with or without digital rectal exam.	Breast self-exam, Clinical breast exam yearly, Screening mammography; Pap Test and HPV test every 3-5 years (discuss with provider); Colonoscopy every 10 years; flexible sigmoidoscopy or virtual colonoscopy every 5 years;
60-70	Colonoscopy every 10 years; flexible sigmoidoscopy or virtual colonoscopy every 5 years; PSA blood test with or without digital rectal exam.	Breast self-exam, Clinical breast exam yearly, Screening mammography (discuss with provider); Pap Test and HPV test every 3-5 years (discuss with provider); Colonoscopy every 10 years; flexible sigmoidoscopy or virtual colonoscopy every 5 years;
70-80	Colonoscopy every 10 years; flexible sigmoidoscopy or virtual colonoscopy every 5 years; PSA blood test with or without digital rectal exam (discuss with provider).	Discuss with provider
80-90	Discuss with provider	Discuss with provider
90-100	Discuss with provider	Discuss with provider

§

References

Fleck, R., & Bach, D. (2012). Trends in Personalized Therapies in Oncology: The (Venture) Capitalist's Perspective. Journal of Personalized Medicine, 2(1), 15-34.

Hirsch, B., & Abernethy, A. (2012). Structured Decision-Making: Using Personalized Medicine to Improve the Value of Cancer Care. Journal of Personalized Medicine, 3(1), 1-13.

Lewis, J., Lipworth, W., & Kerridge, I. (2014). Ethics, Evidence and Economics in the Pursuit of "Personalized Medicine". Journal of Personalized Medicine, 4(2), 137-146.

Royce, T. J., Hendrix, L. H., Stokes, W. A., Allen, I. M., & Chen, R. C. (2014). Cancer screening rates in individuals with different life expectancies. JAMA Intern Med, 174(10), 1558-1565. doi:10.1001/jamainternmed.2014.3895

Verma, M. (2012). Personalized Medicine and Cancer. Journal of Personalized Medicine, 2(1), 1-14.

APPENDIX A1
A TO Z LIST OF CANCER TYPES

A
Acute lymphoblastic leukemia
Acute myeloid leukemia
Adrenocortical carcinoma (adrenal cancer)
Anal cancer
Aplastic anemia
Appendix cancer
Astrocytoma

B
Basal cell carcinoma
Bile duct cancer
Bladder cancer
Bone cancer
Brain stem glioma
Brain/Central Nervous System (CNS) Tumors in Adults
Brain/CNS Tumors in Children
Breast cancer (men and women)

Bronchial tumors
Burkitts lymphoma

C
Carcinoid tumor
Carcinoma of unknown primary
Card tumors
Castleman Disease
Cervical cancer
Chordoma
Chronic lymphocytic leukemia
Chronic myelogenous leukemia
Chronic myeloproliferative disorders
Colon cancer
Colorectal cancer
Craniopharyngioma
Cutaneous T-cell lymphoma

D
Ductal carcinoma in situ

E
Embryonal tumors
Endometrial cancer
Ependymoma
Esophageal cancer
Esthesioneuroblastoma
Ewing Sarcoma (Ewing Family of Tumors)

Extracranial germ cell tumor
Extragonadal germ cell tumor
Extrahepatic bile duct cancer
Eye cancer (intraocular melanoma, retinoblastoma)

G
Gallbladder cancer
Gastric (stomach) cancer
Gastrointestinal carcinoid tumor
Gastrointestinal Stromal Tumors (GIST)
Germ cell tumor (central nervous system, extracranial, extragonadal, ovarian, testicular)
Gestational Trophoblastic tumor
Glioma

H
Hairy cell leukemia
Head and neck cancer
Heart cancer
Hepatocellular (liver) cancer
Histiocytosis, Langerhans Cell
Hodgkins Lymphoma
Hypopharyngeal cancer

I
Intraocular Melanoma
Islet cell Tumor (pancreatic neuroendocrine tumor)

K
Kaposi Sarcoma
Kidney cancer (renal cell, Wilms tumor)

L
Laryngeal and hypopharyngeal cancer
Leukemia (Adults and Children, Acute and Chronic)
Lip and Oral Cavity cancer
Liver cancer (hepatocellular)
Lobular carcinoma in situ (LCIS)
Lung cancer (small cell, non-small cell, carcinoid)

M
Malignant fibrous histiocytoma of bone
Melanoma
Merkel Cell Carcinoma
Mesothelioma
Metastatic Squamous Cell Neck Cancer with Occult Primary
Midline Tract Carcinoma involving NUT Gene
Multiple Endocrine Neoplasia (MEN) syndromes
Multiple Myeloma (Plasma Cell Neoplasm)
Mycosis Fungoides
Myelodysplastic Syndrome

N
Nasal Cavity and Paranasal Sinus Cancer
Nasopharyngeal Cancer

Neuroblastoma
Non-Hodgkins Lymphoma (Adult and Children)

O
Oral Cavity and Oropharyngeal Cancer
Osteosarcoma
Ovarian Cancer

P
Pancreatic Cancer
Penile Cancer
Pituitary Tumors
Prostate Cancer

R
Rectal cancer
Retinoblastoma
Rhabdomyosarcoma

S
Salivary Gland Cancer
Sarcoma (Adult Soft Tissue Cancer)
Sezary Syndrome
Skin Cancer (basal, squamous, melanoma, merkel cell)
Small Cell Lung Cancer
Small Intestine Cancer
Soft Tissue Sarcoma
Squamous Cell Carcinoma

Squamous Neck Cancer with Occult Primary
Stomach Cancer (gastric)

T
T-Cell Lymphoma
Testicular Cancer
Throat Cancer
Thymoma and Thymic Carcinoma
Thyroid Cancer
Transitional Cell Cancer of the Renal Pelvis and Ureter

U
Ureteral Cancer
Uterine Sarcoma

V
Vaginal Cancer
Vulvar Cancer

W
Waldenstrom Macroglobulinemia
Wilms Tumor

Appendix A2
Types of Research Studies

The following types of studies are used to gather information about cancer screening tests:

http://www.cancer.gov/cancertopics/pdq/screening/overview/patient/page6

Randomized controlled trials
Randomized controlled trials give the highest level of evidence about how safe, accurate, and useful cancer screening tests are. In these trials, volunteers are assigned randomly (by chance) to one of two or more groups. The people in one group (the control group) may be given a standard screening test (if one exists) or no screening test. The people in the other group(s) are given the new screening test(s). Test results for the groups are then compared to see if the new screening test works better than the standard test, and to see if there are any harmful side effects.

Using chance to assign people to groups means that the groups will probably be very much alike and that the trial results won't be affected by human choices or something else.

Nonrandomized controlled trials
In nonrandomized clinical trials, volunteers are not assigned randomly (by chance) to different groups. They choose which group they want to be in or the study leaders assign them. Evidence from this type of research is not as strong as evidence from randomized controlled trials.

Cohort studies
A cohort study follows a large number of people over time. The people are divided into groups, called cohorts, based on whether or not they have had a certain treatment or been exposed to certain things. In cohort studies, the information is collected and studied after certain outcomes (such as cancer or death) have occurred. For example, a cohort study might follow a group of women who have regular Pap tests, and divide them into those who test positive for the human papillomavirus (HPV) and those who test negative for HPV. The cohort study would show how the cervical cancer rates are different for the two groups over time.

Case-control studies
Case-control studies are like cohort studies but are done in a shorter time. They do not include many years of

follow-up. Instead of looking forward in time, they look backward. In case-control studies, information is collected from cases (people who already have a certain disease) and compared with information collected from controls (people who do not have the disease). For example, a group of patients with melanoma and a group without melanoma might be asked about how they check their skin for abnormal growths and how often they check it. Based on the different answers from the two groups, the study may show that checking your skin is a useful screening test to decrease the number of melanoma cases and deaths from melanoma.

Evidence from case-control studies is not as strong as evidence from clinical trials or cohort studies.

Ecologic studies
Ecologic studies report information collected on entire groups of people, such as people in one city or county. Information is reported about the whole group, not about any single person in the group. These studies may give some evidence about whether a screening test is useful.

The evidence from ecologic studies is not as strong as evidence from clinical trials or other types of research studies.

APPENDIX A3
FDA APPROVED/CLEARED
COMPANION DIAGNOSTIC
DRUG-DEVICE COMBINATIONS

Table 32. FDA approved/cleared Companion Diagnostic Drug-Device Combinations		
Drug Trade Name	Device Trade Name; Manufacturer	Intended Use; Indications for Use
Erbitux (cetuximab); Vectibix (panitumumab)	DAKO EGFR PharmDx Kit; Dako North America, Inc.	To identify epidermal growth factor receptor (EGFR) expression in normal and neoplastic tissues; Aid in identifying colorectal cancer patients eligible for treatment with named drugs.
Gilotrif (afatinib)	therascreen EGFR RGQ PCR Kit; Qiagen Manchester, Ltd.	Intended to be used to select patients with NSCLC for whom named drug, an EGFR tyrosine kinase inhibitor (TKI), is indicated.
Gleevec/Glivec (imatinib mesylate)	DAKO C-KIT PharmDx; Dako North America, Inc.	Aid in the identification of gastrointestinal stromal tumors (GIST). After diagnosis of GIST, results may be used as an aid in identifying those patients eligible for treatment with named drug.
Herceptin (trastuzumab)	INFORM HER-2/NEU; Ventana Medical Systems, Inc.	Determines the qualitative presence of Her-2/Neu gene amplification; Use as an adjunct to existing clinical and pathologic information currently used as prognostic indicators in the risk stratification of breast cancer in patients who have had a priori invasive, localized breast carcinoma and who are lymph node-negative.
Herceptin (trastuzumab)	PATHVYSION HER-2 DNA Probe Kit; Abbott Molecular Inc	To detect amplification of the HER-2/neu gene; use as an adjunct to existing clinical and pathologic information currently used as prognostic factors in stage II, node-positive breast cancer patients; Aid to predict disease-free and overall survival in patients with stage II, node positive breast cancer treated with adjuvant cyclophosphamide, doxorubicin, and 5-fluorouracil (CAF) chemotherapy; Aid in the assessment of patients for whom named drug is being considered.
Herceptin (trastuzumab)	PATHWAY ANTI-HER-2/NEU (4B5) Rabbit Monoclonal Primary Antibody; Ventana Medical Systems, Inc.	Detection of c-erbB-2 antigen; aid in the assessment of breast cancer patients for whom named drug is being considered.

Herceptin (trastuzumab)	INSITE HER-2/NEU KIT; Biogenex Laboratories, Inc.	Localize the over-expression of Her-2/neu (i.e., c-erbB-2); aid in the assessment of breast cancer patients for whom named drug is being considered.
Herceptin (trastuzumab)	SPOT-LIGHT HER2 CISH Kit; Life Technologies, Inc.	Determine HER2 gene amplification; Aid in the assessment of patients for whom named drug is being considered.
Herceptin (trastuzumab)	Bond Oracle Her2 IHC System; Leica Biosystems	Determine Her2 gene amplification; Aid in the assessment of patients for whom named drug is being considered.
Herceptin (trastuzumab)	HER2 CISH PharmDx Kit; Dako Denmark A/S	Determine HER2 gene status; aid in the assessment of patients for whom named drug is being considered.

§

REFERENCE:

FDA, (2014), List of Cleared or Approved Companion Diagnostic Devices (In Vitro and Imaging Tools), http://www.fda.gov/MedicalDevices/ProductsandMedicalProcedures/InVitroDiagnostics/ucm301431.htm

Appendix A4
FDA Guidance Documents
Related to Personalzed
Medicine

Year Issued	Guidance
2005	Pharmacogenomic Data Submissions
2007	Pharmacogenomic Tests and Genetic Tests for Heritable Markers
2007	Statistical Guidance on Reporting Results from Studies Evaluating Diagnostic Tests
2008	E15 Definitions for Genomic Biomarkers, Pharmacogenomics, Pharmacogenetics, Genomic Data and Sample Coding Categories
2010	Adaptive Design Clinical Trials for Drugs and Biologics (Draft Guidance)
2010	Qualification Process for Drug Development Tools (Draft Guidance)
2011	Clinical Considerations for Therapeutic Cancer Vaccines

2011	Commercially Distributed *In Vitro* Diagnostic Products Labeled for Research Use Only or Investigational Use Only: Frequently Asked Questions (Draft Guidance)
2011	E16 Biomarkers Related to Drug or Biotechnology Product Development: Context, Structure, and Format of Qualification Submissions
2011	Evaluation of Sex Differences in Medical Device Clinical Studies (Draft Guidance)
2011	Applying Human Factors and Usability Engineering to Optimize Medical Device Design (Draft Guidance)
2012	Enrichment Strategies for Clinical Trials to Support Approval of Human Drugs and Biological Products (Draft Guidance)
2012	Factors to Consider When Making Benefit-Risk Determinations in Medical Device Premarket Approval and *De Novo* Classifications
2012	The Content of Investigational Device Exemption (IDE) and Premarket Approval (PMA) Applications for Artificial Pancreas Device Systems
2013	Mobile Medical Applications
2013	Clinical Pharmacogenomics: Premarket Evaluation in Early-Phase Clinical Studies and Recommendations for Labeling
2013	FDA Decisions for Investigational Device Exemption (IDE) Clinical Investigations (Draft Guidance)[19]
2013	Molecular Diagnostic Instruments with Combined Functions (Draft Guidance)

2013	Providing Information about Pediatric Uses of Medical Devices Under Section 515A of the Federal Food, Drug, and Cosmetic Act (Draft Guidance)
2013	Submissions for Postapproval Modifications to a Combination Product Approved Under a BLA, NDA, or PMA (Draft Guidance)
2013	Current Good Manufacturing Requirements for Combination Products Final Rule
2014	*In Vitro* Companion Diagnostic Devices - Guidance for Industry and FDA Staff

FDA, (2014) Select FDA Guidance Documents That Relate to Personalized Medicine, http://www.fda.gov/ScienceResearch/SpecialTopics/PersonalizedMedicine/ucm372544.htm

Appendix A5
Additional Resources

Cancer Care

Books
Laughlin, E.H *Coming to Terms with Cancer: A Glossary of Cancer-Related Terms Easily Understood*, 2nd Edition, ISBN: 1484908228

Greco, K.E., Tinley, S., & Seibert, D. (2012). *Essential Genetic and Genomic Competencies for Nurses with Graduate Degrees.* Silver Spring, MD: American Nurses Association and International Society of Nurses in Genetics

Journal Issues
Seminars in Oncology Nursing, Volume 30. No. 2 "Personalizing Patient Care with Precision Medicine" www.nursongoncology.com

Websites
American Cancer Society http://www.cancer.org/

American Institute for Cancer Research http://www.aicr.org/

American Society for Clinical Oncology http://www.cancer.net/

America Society of Human Genetics http://www.ashg.org

American Society for Therapeutic Radiology and Oncology http://www.astro.org

Association of Cancer Online Resources http://www.acor.org/

Cancer at Medline Plus http://www.nlm.nih.gov/medlineplus/cancer.html

Cancer Care http://www.cancercare.org/

Cancer Hope Network http://www.cancerhopenetwork.org/
Consortium of Academic Health Centers for Integrative Medicine http://www.imconsortium.org/

International Society of Nurses in Genetics http://www.isong.org

Livestrong Foundation http://www.livestrong.org/

MD Anderson Cancer Center http://www.mdanderson.org/patient-and-cancer-information/index.html

National Cancer Institute http://www.cancer.gov/

National Center for Complementary and Alternative Medicine http://nccam.nih.gov/

National Comprehensive Cancer Network http://www.nccn.org/

National Institutes of Health: Genetic and Rare Diseases Information Center www.rarediseases.info.nih.gov/gard

National Society of Genetic Counselors http://www.nsgc.org

Oncology Nursing Society http://www.ons.org

University of Pennsylvania http://www.oncolink.org/

CANCER RISK ASSESSMENT TOOLS
NCI Breast Cancer Risk Assessment Tool www.cancer.gov/bcrisktool

NCI Colorectal Cancer Risk Assessment Tool www.cancer.gov/colorectalcancerrisk

COMPLEMENTARY AND ALTERNATIVE MEDICINE

Databases
National Medicines Comprehensive Database http://hprc-online.org/dietary-supplements/natural-medicines-comprehensive-database

National Standard Databases https://naturalmedicines.therapeuticresearch.com/databases/

Websites
American Botanical Council http://abc.herbalgram.org/site/PageServer

American Cancer Society

- Complementary and Alternative Medicine http://www.cancer.org/treatment/treatmentsandsideeffects/complementaryandalternativemedicine/index
- Guidelines for Using Complementary and Alternative Methods http://www.cancer.org/treatment/treatmentsandsideeffects/complementaryandalternativemedicine/guidelines-for-using-complementary-and-alternative-methods

American Herbal Product Association http://ahpa.org/
Food and Drug Administration

- Buying Medicines and Medical Products Online http://www.fda.gov/ForConsumers/ProtectYourSelf/default.htm
- Center for Food Safety and Applied Nutrition: Dietary Supplements http://www.fda.gov/Food/DietarySupplements/default.htm
- Consumer Updates http://www.fda.gov/ForConsumers/ConsumerUpdates/default.htm

National Institutes of Health

National Library of Medicine http://www.nlm.nih.gov

- CAM on PubMed® http://nccam.nih.gov/research/camonpubmed
- Dietary Supplement Label Database http://www.dsld.nlm.nih.gov/dsld

Medline Plus

- MedlinePlus Herbs and Supplements http://www.nlm.nih.gov/medlineplus/druginformation.html
- MedlinePlus Complementary and Alternative Medicine Page http://www.nlm.nih.gov/medlineplus/complementaryandalternativemedicine.html

National Cancer Institute (NCI) http://www.cancer.gov

- NCI PDQ® Cancer Information Summaries: Complementary and Alternative Medicine http://www.cancer.gov/cancertopics/pdq/cam
- NCI PDQ® Cancer Information Summaries: Supportive and Palliative Care (Coping With Cancer) http://www.cancer.gov/cancertopics/pdq/supportivecare

National Center for Complementary and Alternative Medicine (NCCAM) http://nccam.nih.gov/health

- Health Topics A-Z http://nccam.nih.gov/health/atoz.htm
- Herbs at a Glance http://nccam.nih.gov/health/herbsataglance.htm – complete list may be downloaded as a free e-book
- Clinical Practice Guidelines http://nccam.nih.gov/health/providers/clinicalpractice.htm

Office of Dietary Supplements Fact Sheets http://ods.od.nih.gov/Health_Information/Information_About_Individual_Dietary_Supplements.aspx

Society for Integrative Oncology http://www.integrativeonc.org/

About the Author

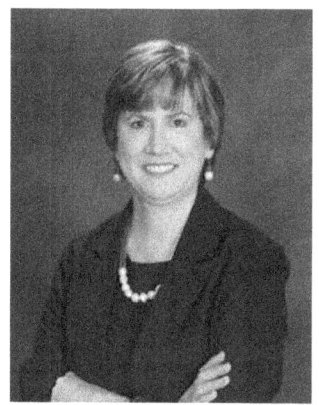

Colleen Lee is a board certified nurse practitioner, clinical nurse specialist and founder of Lee Medical Case Review, LLC (lee-medical.com), a legal nurse consulting company assisting clients in medically-related cases. As an author of award-winning journal articles, book chapters, and web courses on cancer treatment and symptom management, Lee is also the co-author of *"Cancer and*

Complementary Medicine: Your Guide to Smart Choices in Symptom Management," an informative text for making safe choices surrounding cancer treatment.

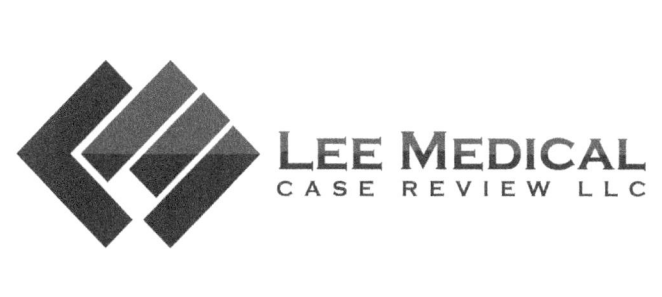

www.ingramcontent.com/pod-product-compliance
Lightning Source LLC
Chambersburg PA
CBHW071712170526
45165CB00005B/1985